Chronic respiratory illness

T0173818

Chronic obstructive airways disease (COAD: bronchitis, emphysema and chronic asthma) is a major medical, psychological, social and economic problem. Breathlessness is one of the most distressing and disabling symptoms of COAD, and it has long been apparent that the condition results in impaired quality of life.

Drawing upon sociological and psychological sources, and his own detailed research within this area, Simon Williams sensitively portrays the meaning, experience and impact of COAD. Sufferers' and their families' own accounts are used to portray the various stages and aspects of COAD, ranging from the experience of symptoms and the management of medical regimens, to the practical problems it creates in daily life and the more diffuse and intangible ways in which it impinges upon social and family life. He also provides a comprehensive review of the relevant psychosocial literature and concludes by discussing some of the policy implications for health care professionals.

Chronic Respiratory Illness will be of immense value to health professionals and others who care for sufferers and their families. It will also be of interest to students and researchers working in medical sociology, health psychology, medicine and nursing.

Simon J. Williams is Lecturer in Sociology at the University of Warwick.

The Experience of Illness

Series Editors: Ray Fitzpatrick and Stanton Newman

Chronic respiratory illness

Simon J. Williams

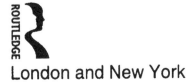

London and New York

First published 1993
by Routledge
11 New Fetter Lane, London EC4P 4EE

Simultaneously published in the USA and Canada
by Routledge
29 West 35th Street, New York, NY 10001

© 1993 Simon J. Williams

Typeset in Times by
NWL Editorial Services, Langport, Somerset

Transferred to digital printing 2003

British Library Cataloguing in Publication Data
A catalogue record for this book is available from the British
Library.

Library of Congress Cataloging in Publication Data
Williams, Simon (Simon Johnson), 1961–
  Chronic respiratory illness / Simon Williams.
  p.   cm. – (The Experience of illness)
  Includes bibliographical references and index.
  1. Lungs – Diseases, Obstructive – Psychological aspects.
  2. Lungs – Diseases, Obstructive – Social aspects.
  I. Title.   II. Series.
  RC776.03W55   1993   92–39592
  362.1'962 – dc20   CIP

ISBN 0–415–07657–9

Contents

Editors' preface

Chronic respiratory disorders are a major source of distress and disability for sufferers and their families. They are among the large class of human illnesses in which the relationship between underlying physiological indices and symptomatic severity is only weak. This is prima-facie evidence that personal meaning and social context have a major influence on the experience of respiratory problems. As Simon Williams points out, breathing is a fundamental function that we take for granted; when it is disturbed, for whatever reason, it may constitute the most distressing of experiences.

Simon Williams has provided us with a unique account of the lives of individuals who experience respiratory problems. His study is based on detailed investigation of a sample of sufferers' experiences using both standardised quantitative measures of impairment, disability and handicap, as well as in-depth interviews. The result is a remarkably well-observed and sensitive analysis of respiratory disorders as viewed by sufferers. It is vital to be reminded of the scope for improving individuals' quality of life. The author makes a powerful case for those who would see important challenges surrounding the task of improving the daily lives of people with chronic illnesses. The first stage of this task is to be fully aware of the true impact of illness. Work such as this book is central in displaying graphically the burden of illness which sufferers, carers, families and health services confront.

Ray Fitzpatrick and Stanton Newman, 1993

Author's preface

The main source upon which this book draws is a detailed study, by the author, of the consequences of chronic respiratory illness (Chronic Obstructive Airways Disease – COAD), focusing particularly on the meaning, experience, impact (i.e. physical, psychological, social, economic and material) and management of the condition. This involved both a detailed and systematic *quantitative* investigation of these issues with a sample of ninety-two COAD out-patients, and further in-depth, *qualitative*, tape-recorded, domiciliary interviews with a smaller sub-sample of twenty-four sufferers and, wherever possible, their carers. It is the latter, qualitative data source upon which this book principally relies for insights into the meaning, experience, impact and management of COAD, for both sufferers and their families. Further details of the study are to be found in Williams (1990), and Williams and Bury (1989a, b).

It should be emphasised at the outset that this is *not* primarily a book about the experience of asthma, the study of which represents a separate, yet related, issue. Rather, as Chapter one explains, the population of COAD sufferers tends to be predominantly composed of those with chronic obstructive bronchitis and emphysema. Only those cases of chronic asthma where the obstruction has, over a period of time usually spanning many years, become less *reversible* may be subsumed under this rubric.

I would like to thank Mike Bury, my Ph.D. supervisor, for his help, encouragement, guidance and support over the years; Mike Calnan and everyone else at the Centre for Health Services Studies, University of Kent, who have made the time I spent writing this book so enjoyable; the editors, Ray Fitzpatrick and Stanton Newman, for offering me the chance to write a book for the series, and to Ray in particular for his general support and encouragement over the years; Dr Robin Rudd and his colleagues for help in actually setting up the study and allowing me access to their patients; and also, of course, the patients themselves and their families, who gave of their time so generously despite the stress and strains they, undoubtedly, were under. Needless to say, the names of all individuals referred to within the book have been changed in order to preserve confidentiality.

Thanks also go to Gill Bendelow, Sarah Cant, Alicia Deale and Pete and Fran Cuthbert, for help, encouragement and support. Last, but certainly not least, thanks must also go to my parents, to whom I undoubtedly owe the greatest debt of all. This book is dedicated to them both.

Chapter 1

Chronic obstructive airways disease
Clinical nature and epidemiology

Chronic obstructive airways disease (COAD: emphysema, chronic obstructive bronchitis and chronic asthma) is a 'debilitating disease of adult life'. Despite differences of opinion amongst pulmonary physicians as to the precise definition of COAD, the term has nevertheless enjoyed common usage within the medical literature for approximately twenty-five years and most would agree that the cardinal feature is one of expiratory obstruction to airflow (McSweeny and Labuhn 1990).

COAD is a major, though neglected, medical and social problem in the United Kingdom today. Indeed, it is one of the leading causes of absence from work in the UK (OHE 1977), and it has long been apparent that COAD results in impaired quality of life. As Capel and Caplin state, COAD 'maims before it kills' (1964: 16). Dyspnoea (breathlessness) is one of the most distressing (Hinton 1967) and disabling (Lane 1988) symptoms of COAD. As Hinton notes: 'The breathlessness experienced by those with slowly encroaching disease of the lungs is not easily relieved' (1967: 80). Indeed, the ability to breathe is the *sine qua non* of life. Consequently, 'an elemental fear is soon aroused' (Hinton 1967). Although the mechanisms of breathlessness are poorly understood, there is a growing body of evidence to suggest that psychosocial factors are implicated, even when severe lung disease is present (Rosser and Guz 1981, Jones 1988). Furthermore, the fact that COAD in the UK disproportionately affects those from working-class backgrounds (Townsend *et al.* 1988), who may well be least able to cope with its consequences (i.e. the fact that it is 'socially patterned': MacIntyre 1986, 1988), adds a further dimension of disadvantage to both sufferers and their families.

THE CLINICAL NATURE OF COAD

In 1808 Charles Badham adopted the term 'bronchitis' to define collectively 'chronic pectoral (chest) complaints, especially those of people advanced in life' (OHE 1977). However, through an intriguing history of shifting terminology and conceptual acrobatics (Scadding 1981), we have now arrived at the term *chronic obstructive airways disease* (COAD) – or something similar such as *chronic obstructive pulmonary disease* (COPD), or *chronic airflow limitation* (CAL). COAD is a rather broad catch-all term which encompasses chronic obstructive bronchitis, emphysema and, although there does not seem to be any consensus here, certain cases of chronic asthma, in recognition of the fact that these conditions often co-exist.

The Medical Research Council Committee on the Aetiology of Chronic Bronchitis considered the issue of terminology in 1965. They accepted that the criteria for emphysema should be defined in morbid-anatomical terms. They suggested that the term 'chronic bronchitis', which was by now firmly entrenched in British clinical usage, should be retained with formal definitions, primarily in clinical-descriptive terms (Scadding 1981). Thus, chronic bronchitis may be defined as the 'occurrence of cough and phlegm on most days for at least three months in the year for two successive years' (MRC 1965: 775). Chronic bronchitis is often complicated by recurrent chest illness and may be associated with airflow obstruction leading to breathlessness on exertion, in which case it is referred to as chronic *obstructive* bronchitis. Emphysema often co-exists.

Emphysema may be said to be present where there is 'enlargement of airspaces beyond the terminal non-respiratory bronchioles, usually with destruction of lung tissue' (RCP 1981). These changes, which are usually caused by very fine penetrations of smoke, dust or other substances of a noxious nature, lead to a loss of the lungs' natural elasticity (recoil) which results in the lungs tending to be permanently inflated. As the Royal College of Physicians' (RCP) report points out:

> The diagnosis covers a range of types of abnormality which can only be identified with certainty by pathological examination. The main symptom is breathlessness on exertion and this is associated with changes in lung function which may take a characteristic form. However, where chronic bronchitis co-exists it is seldom possible to separate their respective contributions to respiratory disability.
>
> (1981: 70)

Finally, asthma is characterised, in contrast to chronic obstructive bronchitis and emphysema, by 'obstruction to airflow which is *variable* spontaneously and in response to treatment. However, over a period of time, which is usually measured in years, the obstruction may become less reversible' (RCP 1981: 70). Thus, whilst the majority of asthma sufferers are not included under the rubric of COAD, those chronic asthmatics whose airflow obstruction has, over time, become less revisible may be subsumed under this general term.

Hence the term COAD refers to those respiratory conditions characterised by abnormally high resistance to airflow in intrapulmonary airways. This may be due to changes of various sorts in the airways themselves or to emphysema, or to a combination of these. Consequently, the term 'airflow obstruction' has been used rather widely and loosely to refer to this abnormality of function (Scadding 1981). This is usually diagnosed when the degree of fixed obstruction results in a 'Forced Expiratory Volume in one second (FEV_1) less than 70 per cent of predicted values' for age, sex and height (Guyatt *et al.* 1987). Thus defined, the population of COAD sufferers tends to be predominantly composed of those with chronic obstructive bronchitis and emphysema, together with a small proportion of chronic asthma suffers whose obstruction has become progressively less revisible over time.

As mentioned above, the predominant and most distressing symptom is that of breathlessness on exertion (dyspnoea), which is frequently accompanied by a chronic cough and excessive mucus production. In addition, in certain more advanced cases, oxygen deficiencies (hypoxaemia) and/or excessive carbon dioxide retention (hypercapnia) in the blood (i.e. blood gas abnormalities) are to be found – which may result in neuro-psychological dysfunction (Prigatano and Grant 1988) – together with decreased cardiac efficiency and right-sided heart failure (cor pulmonale). Consequently, eventual death results.

It is not within the scope of this chapter to go into existing research on possible causal factors in the aetiology of such conditions. However, suffice it to say that the contribution of factors such as the following: cigarette smoking (Fletcher *et al.* 1976) – itself class-linked (Blaxter 1987, 1990); air pollution (Colley *et al.* 1970, 1973); occupation (Hunter 1975); housing and material conditions (Holma and Kjaer 1980, Burr *et al.* 1981); and early childhood experience (Kiernan *et al.* 1976, Britten *et al.* 1987), is now well established. In addition certain hereditary genetic factors appear to modify susceptibility – the key one being an $alpha_1$-antitrypsin deficiency. However, of all these factors, Petty (1985) has suggested that COAD would be a relatively minor health problem if people did not smoke.

Despite considerable uncertainty concerning the early natural history of COAD, it is now widely accepted that it begins at a relatively early stage in life and is characterised by a slowly progressive, insidious, deterioration of lung function for many years prior to the development and presentation of frank clinical illness (Burrows 1985). The perception of COAD on the patient's part is, of course, subject to various social and cultural determinants, such that onset rarely coincides with the subjective perception and presentation of symptoms. However, it remains possible that COAD can have a fairly abrupt onset, with a rapid decrease in ventilatory capacity occurring during the few years prior to the onset of symptoms (Burrows 1985).

The subsequent course of the disease following the development of significant symptomatology is considerably better documented and understood. As Burrows notes:

> In general patients become unable to perform very vigorous exertion once their FEV_1 falls much below 1.5 litres, but are often able to continue work, unless their job is very physically demanding, until their FEV_1 falls below 1.0 litres. However, there is considerable variability in the relationship of impairment to disability, some of which appears to relate to psychological factors.

(1985: 37)

The degree of disability accompanying COAD may usefully be classified according to the following five levels of functioning:

1 Patient with recognised disease but with *no* restriction: is able to do what peers can do and continues usual life style.
2 Patient with *minimally* restricted activity who is able to do productive work: has some difficulty keeping up with peers and has begun to modify life style.
3 Patient with *moderately* restricted activity: is not homebound but may not be able to do productive work, however still able to care for him/herself.
4 Patient with *markedly* restricted activity: limited outdoor mobility, unable to do productive work but is still able to care for him/herself, albeit with difficulty.
5 Patient with *very severely* restricted activity: is essentially/totally housebound, needs help with personal care/is unable to care for him/herself. (Adapted from the American Lung Association 1975.)

Concerning longevity, Burrows finds that 'median survival is approximately 10 years when the FEV_1 is 1.4 litres, approaches 4 years when FEV_1 has fallen to 1.0 litres and is little more than 2 years when the FEV_1 nears 500 millilitres' (1985: 37–8). The medical treatment and management of COAD is discussed in Chapter three.

THE EPIDEMIOLOGY OF COAD

Bronchitis, emphysema and asthma, amongst other respiratory conditions, are major contributors to the national pool of chronic illness and disability in the United Kingdom. International comparisons of mortality rates from such conditions indicate quite clearly that they affect the UK populace to a far greater extent than any other country in the world (OHE 1977). As the Office of Health Economics (OHE) report states: 'Mortality in the UK from all chronic lung conditions during the mid 1960's was probably in the order of 10 times that experienced in Japan, Sweden and Norway and several times that which occurred in most other industrialised countries' (1977: 18). In the United States of America, the prevalence rate in 1980 was 4.75 per cent, and COAD accounted for approximately 2.5 per cent of all deaths – thus ranking as the fifth leading cause of mortality (Tockman *et al.* 1985). However, at least some of these international differences could partly be explained by the different usage of terminology (e.g. the difference between the frequently used clinical diagnosis of emphysema in the United States and the predominantly pathological diagnosis adopted in the United Kingdom at autopsy). Furthermore, as mentioned earlier, mortality rates for diseases of the respiratory system, such as bronchitis, show extremely steep social class gradients which have been in existence throughout the twentieth century. Whilst concerning morbidity, a survey of 92 GPs distributed throughout the country found that the percentage of men and women between the ages of 40 and 60 who were suffering from chronic bronchitis rose sharply with descending social class from 6 per cent in class I to 26 per cent in class V (Townsend *et al.* 1988).

A useful source of data is to be found in the Royal College of Physicians' (RCP) report on disabling chest disease (1981). According to the report, in 1976/7 the number of person-days lost from work due to bronchitis, chronic bronchitis and emphysema was in the order of 26 million for men and 2.6 million for women; constituting approximately 10 per cent of all recorded working days lost due to sickness absence. The cost of sickness benefit, if expressed at current rates, was somewhat in excess of 100 million, and the total economic cost to the community considerably more. As the RCP report states: 'The associated load on the GP service was reflected in the GP consultations of which, in 1971, 21 per cent were on account of respiratory ill-health including infections of the upper and lower respiratory tracts' (1981: 71).

The numbers suffering from chronic respiratory illness and disability are also reflected in the figures for invalidity benefit and for those who are in receipt of non-contributory invalidity pension. In 1977, approximately 68,000 men of working age and 6,000 women were in receipt of these benefits as a result of chronic respiratory illness, whilst in 1978 the Disabled Persons' Register, admittedly a poor measure of disability in the community, included some 57,000 entries as a result of respiratory disability (RCP 1981). As the RCP report states:

> if it assumed that the number of chronically sick constitute a similar proportion of the national pool of such persons then the total number of men of working age with respiratory impairment sufficient to make them potential candidates for invalidity benefit is of the order of 0.3 million.
>
> (1981: 71)

This figure is consistent with certain epidemiological evidence concerning the prevalence of chronic bronchitis in the community (e.g. 25 per cent amongst men aged 50–9 years: Fletcher *et al.* 1976).

However, disability, of course, varies considerably in terms of its degree of severity. Thus in Harris *et al.*'s survey of the 'handicapped and impaired in Great Britain' (1971), the actual number of individuals with a respiratory disorder who required help with some item of daily living was estimated to be about 20,000. Above working age about twice this number were found to be similarly disabled (Harris *et al.* 1971). A further indication of severe disability can be found in the figures for attendance and mobility allowances. As the RCP report states:

> at the end of 1978 there were 7,600 persons with chronic respiratory disease on whose behalf an attendance allowance was being paid; 6,000 being cases of bronchitis. In October 1979 mobility allowance was being paid to some 4,209 persons aged 60 years or less disabled by chronic lung disease.
>
> (1981: 71)

A more recent estimate by the Office of Population Censuses and Surveys (OPCS 1988a), suggests that of the just over 6 million disabled adults living in Great Britain today, 13 per cent of those living in private households and 6 per cent of those living in communal establishments suffer from diseases of the respiratory system.

The figures for previous years indicate that the number of persons receiving sickness benefit or invalidity benefit for bronchitis has remained relatively stable. In contrast, the number of hospital admissions on account of chronic bronchitis and emphysema has been steadily declining, as has the associated mortality rate, which rises with age (RCP 1981). However, mortality rates attributable to such conditions convey a somewhat distorted picture as the condition is rarely fatal in middle life; around four-fifths of all deaths occurring in people aged 65 or over. Hence death from the condition usually occurs only after years of progressively worsening disability and suffering (OHE 1977). On average, approximately 10 per cent of hospital beds throughout the year are occupied by chest cases, of whom about half are chronic bronchitics, with the proportion rising steeply in the winter months (RCP 1981). The picture is generally similar for men and women, although fewer women are affected. The cost to the NHS of treating such conditions is enormous; estimates indicate that in 1974, for example, the treatment of bronchitis and emphysema cost the NHS approximately 95 million (OHE 1977). As the RCP report (1981) notes, for a variety of reasons, ranging from problems surrounding actual clinical diagnosis to the measurement of disability, the above figures are inevitably of limited reliability and validity. However, the biasing factors do not all operate in a similar direction and so, when taken together, they confirm that the extent of respiratory disablement, and the management and support of those suffering such conditions, present us with major problems both in terms of human suffering and misery, and in terms of the demands placed upon health and welfare services and the community as a whole.

Having sketched a brief clinical and epidemiological picture of COAD, it is to a more detailed discussion of the *experiential* and *subjective* dimensions of its symptomatology that the next chapter now turns.

Chapter 2

The subjective experience and management of symptoms

There are certain common themes which are to be found running through the lives of all those who suffer a chronic, disabling disorder. Thus perennial problems of work, income, social and family life are frequently mentioned dimensions of experience by those who suffer any sort of chronic, disabling condition regardless of its nature. However, there are certain other problems which, as Locker states, 'are not common to all those with a chronic disorder since they originate in the nature of the particular impairment and the way it manifests itself in symptoms' (1983: 14).

Indeed there are important facets and dimensions of COAD symptomatology which make the experience of living with the illness substantially different from other chronic conditions. Thus, as Fagerhaugh (1975) suggests, emphysema sufferers are constantly having to contend with disabling breathlessness and a reduced oxygen supply, which involves a strategy of selectively allocating their diminished supplies of what she terms 'basic mobility resources' (BMRs), such as time, energy and money. As Strauss (1975) has argued, experiencing and learning how to manage the disruptive, often distressing, nature of the symptoms created by the disease is an important part of the *experience* of living with a chronic illness on a daily basis. Indeed, as Locker states:

> the early stages of the disabled person's career may consist entirely of a process of learning to cope with and adapt to the symptoms of the disease itself rather than the wider social consequences that follow appreciable disability. In this respect, the biological realities that constitute disease, though mediated by individual and societal responses, have an important impact on an individual's daily life and life chances.
>
> (1983: 14)

Hence this chapter provides a detailed discussion of the practical, experiential and cognitive problems which the *symptoms* of COAD themselves create, together with the manner in which they are managed or handled within the context of sufferers' daily lives.

THE ONSET OF CHRONIC RESPIRATORY DISORDER

In the short term the onset of chronic illness may be conceptualised as a 'critical incident'; one which disrupts and throws into relief taken-for-granted assumptions regarding the past, present and future. This results in considerable uncertainty and calls for some sort of explanatory framework which will endow this *biographically disruptive* phenomenon with a semblance of meaning (Bury 1982). As Sontag (1978) remarks: 'illness rarely knocks before it enters'. In the longer term, as Locker states, 'it results in a reduction of physical resources so that mundane practical matters of everyday life can no longer be taken-for-granted but become problems that need to be solved' (1983: 5–6).

As discussed in Chapter one, the predominant pattern of COAD tends to be of a relatively slow and insidious onset, often over the course of many years, with symptoms initially either being ignored or 'explained away' in less serious or threatening terms. In most cases, the primary initial symptom which gives rise to a recognition that something is wrong is the experience of breathlessness on exertion – although chronic coughing, recurrent (winter) chest infections, together with general feelings of tiredness, lethargy and of 'slowing down', are also often mentioned. For example, in Williams' (1990) study of COAD, sufferers often struggled to date onset precisely, and the initial onset of symptoms did not always lead to an immediate medical consultation; symptoms frequently being 'explained away' in other less threatening terms. Indeed, there was often a considerable time-lag between the initial perception of symptoms, their being taken 'seriously', and their subsequent medical presentation, and it seemed that often it was only retrospectively that the 'obvious' or 'self-evident' character of the symptoms and what they symbolised was recognised. That is to say, it was only with hindsight that they became self-evident or obvious manifestations of COAD. It is within such contexts that issues of uncertainty and the legitimacy of symptoms loom large. Tentative ideas, beliefs and modes of explanation are constantly having to be revised in the light of new evidence as the illness unfolds. In addition, individuals are faced with difficult choices regarding the strategic social management of symptoms: namely, the dilemma of whether to display or disclose one's symptoms (Bury 1988).

Thus Mr O'Riley, a scaffolder by trade, described the onset of his condition and his initial reaction to it in the following manner:

I first noticed it about, oh, I s'pose roughly about 12 years back now. . . . Yeah roughly about 12 years back when I noticed it. But it must have been building up prior to that, but, ah, I didn't know about it, you know. In my job see, it was all climbing up and down, I could climb anything. But then I seemed to slow down . . . I didn't take much notice of it at the time, at that time I thought it was just because I was getting older and all that, you know. . . . 'Cause you don't expect to be able to do what an 18 year old can do at that age do you?

Consequently, he delayed doing anything about it for quite a considerable period of time:

No I didn't do nothing at first. You see, because there was a simple reason why: I didn't think it was serious. I didn't think it was anything serious. Because I was smoking, and a lot of people, well, you know, you get a bit of a cough and all that with smoking don't you, you know, a smoker's cough and what have you. And so you put it down to the smoking and all that, just cut back a bit, you know. 'Cause I must admit I was a heavy smoker, I do admit that.

In a similar vein, Mrs Cole retrospectively dated onset as being approximately ten years prior to interview. However, she claimed she had really only started to take notice of it in within the last couple of years or so since it had begun to interfere considerably with her life, forcing her to give up work:

Well, before I sort of got as bad as this I used to get a bit breathless, you know, when I used to run a bit, for a bus or something like that. But that sort of breathlessness, well that's different in'it, it was explainable, understandable, d'you know what I mean. You *felt* all right like, and you didn't take much notice of it anyway sort of thing. But now, well, you couldn't run with this, with it like it is now. It feels sort of different from a normal shortness of breath, from when you've been running or something like that. It's sort of different, it isn't normal is it. It's when it gets to that stage that, really, you start to sit up and take notice of it sort of thing, you know. You can't just put it down to having over-exerted yourself, gettin' older, being a bit out of shape, just a smoker's cough or what have you. It's then you realise it's more than that, that something's really wrong with you like.

Similarly Cornwell (1984), in her study of health and illness in East

London, found that respondents tended to classify certain common respiratory diseases as 'normal' illnesses, or 'health problems that are not illnesses', rather than being 'real' illness. As the illness became progressively more disabling, however, there was a transition or re-classification of the symptoms as manifestations of 'real' illness which legitimately fell within the province of medicine and warranted medical attention.

THE SYMPTOMATIC CHARACTER AND EXPERIENCE OF LIVING WITH COAD

Breathlessness

The etymon of the term dyspnoea can be traced right back to Ancient Greece where it was used quite literally to refer to 'ill-breathing' or 'bad breathing' (Petty and Nett 1984). As one may perhaps expect, dyspnoea tends to be the predominant, most distressing and disabling symptom experienced by COAD sufferers. Indeed, in Williams' (1990) study for example, sufferers often spoke of their breathlessness and medical condition as being synonymous. Thus being breathless meant having emphysema or chronic bronchitis, just as having emphysema or chronic bronchitis meant being breathless: a case quite literally of the two being spoken of in the same 'breath'. As Fagerhaugh states:

> The mobility problem of the emphysema victim is primarily one of inability to get enough oxygen to produce energy. A certain amount of energy is necessary to maintain the body at rest; for physical activity a [lung] oxygen reserve volume is required. Depending upon the activity, more or less oxygen is necessary. In advanced emphysema, because of pathological changes, there is very limited oxygen reserve, and maintaining the reserve is difficult. These patients become short of breath with minimal physical activity, and compared to 'normal lungers' require longer and more frequent periods to 'recoup' their diminished oxygen reserve.

Moreover:

> Adequate lung reserve is necessary not only for physical mobility, but for such vocalizations as talking, laughing, singing or yelling. . . . Because of advanced stages of emphysema, extended talking, laughing, or crying can trigger off paroxysms of coughing as well as respiratory distress.

(1975: 100–1)

Despite the objective variability in the level of breathlessness actually experienced by those in Williams' (1990) study, 82 per cent perceived it as a 'big problem' in their daily lives. As noted in Chapter one, when one's breathing is affected an 'elemental fear is soon aroused' (Hinton 1967). Perhaps not surprisingly then, many sufferers tended to experience bouts of fear or panic when breathless. The following accounts, starting with that of Mr King, convey something of the frightening experience when gripped by a sudden attack of breathlessness:

> Well of course the major symptom is the *breathlessness*. Sometimes it's terribly, terribly bad, I get so short of breath that any inhaler is no good, you just have to sit down and pray it passes. The last thing in the world you want to do is to get excited or panic about it, because when you do, you get so far out of breath that you put yourself in an absolutely desperate situation. You just have to sit down and try and remain calm until your breath comes back. It's a very frightening thing to have to live with because *it threatens your very existence*, or at least you feel that it does when it strikes. But as I say, you've just gotta try and stay calm, it's not easy but it's essential, because if you don't, boy you're in even bigger trouble. . . . It's very difficult not to panic when you're gasping for breath, simply because you don't know if you're ever going to be able to draw another breath! This is the way it is, you get to that kind of situation that, well you think to yourself: 'Am I ever going to be able to pull in another inhalation?' You look at it like that. It puts you in a desperate situation altogether. You're quite literally fighting for your life.

Mr Ash, meanwhile, remarked:

> Well there are stages of breathlessness. For instance, I could be sitting here, and just from getting up and walking outside, I'd be out of breath. Then I'll have to slow down a little bit or stop and get me breath back. Then I'll walk upstairs and I'll come to the next stage of getting out of breath, where I've gotta go on the oxygen by the time I reach the top. I have to sit on the bed for a while with the oxygen on. Then I'll go a stage further when I just seem to get out of breath all of a sudden like, you know, it'll come on in a spasm, a sudden attack, or I'll over-do it a bit. You know, I'll frighten meself I'll be so breathless, I'm literally fighting for me breath then. When I get out of breath like that I seem to get more and more frightened, you start to panic, you can't stop yourself, you can't help it, you do panic.
>   . . . it's very frightening, you must panic, you've gotta panic when

you get like that, you're in a desperate situation, dire straits. Well, to tell you the truth, once I was upstairs and I was so breathless that I ended up sitting on the toilet banging me head into me hands. Honestly, I was so panicky and short of breath, I was desperate. But generally, I was told a long time ago to make meself count, to try and concentrate on counting, you know, count on breathing in and count on breathing out. They say it's supposed to take your mind off the breathing and help you to regain control, and so I've always done that, it's sort of second nature now, a natural thing to turn to, you know. I mean I might be out of breath and panicky, but I still try to make meself count, 'cause I find it helps.

Finally, Mrs McLeod spoke of her experience concerning sudden attacks of breathlessness in the following terms:

It's very frightening, I can't speak, I can't move, I'm just like a statue, you know. If I was out on my own I couldn't call for help or anything like that, I'm just like a statue, frozen stiff with fear. And you begin to break out into a cold, sickly, sweat. You're gasping for air, and you feel as if you're suffocating, as if a vacuum is sucking the air right out of you, you know. Oh, I can't tell you what it's like really, it's just very, very frightening. To be honest with you, when you're like that, you get into such a panic you don't know what's happening to you really, it's terrible.

These accounts illustrate quite graphically the 'elemental fear' aroused when breathing is undermined, and its potentially crippling nature both physically and mentally. As mentioned in Chapter one, the ability to breathe is the *sine qua non* of life. Indeed, as Mr King's account suggests, when in the grips of a sudden, frightening attack, sufferers often subjectively felt that they were locked into a battle for life; for their very existence. Hence, fear and panic are perhaps understandable responses. Some also spoke with a sense of humiliation and shame, of actually losing control of their bladders in the event of a bad attack, and thus of wetting themselves. Yet if the experience of breathlessness seems formidable enough, the reality of COAD and its associated symptomatology means having to cope with more than just this. Hence, it is to a discussion of these further dimensions of symptomatology that this chapter now turns.

Other dimensions of symptomatology

COAD is a multifaceted disease. In a novel approach, Kinsman and his colleagues (1983) constructed a checklist of eighty-nine symptoms which

COAD patients commonly experience. Similarly, Guyatt *et al.* (1987) devised a 108-item questionnaire in order to determine the frequency and importance of all significant areas of dysfunction in COAD. In both studies problems of dyspnoea and fatigue frequently occurred, whilst cognitive impairment appeared to be a less important dimension of experience. Sleep difficulties were found to be more prominent in Kinsman *et al.*'s study, whilst items concerning embarrassment, anxiety and depression were not only more frequently reported, but also rated with a higher degree of importance in Guyatt *et al.*'s patients. However, caution is needed here in making such comparisons, as Kinsman *et al.*'s study contained a sample of 149 hospitalised patients, whilst Guyatt *et al.*'s was of 100 out-patients and excluded 24 'severe' cases.

As mentioned above, one of the predominant characteristics of COAD is a generalised lack of energy, coupled with a constant feeling of tiredness and lethargy due to an inability to get enough oxygen to furnish one's energy requirements (Fagerhaugh 1975). Thus, in Williams' (1990) study, for example, the majority of sufferers found a lack of energy a problem in their daily lives. As Mrs White put it:

> Oh I get very tired very easily. I mean I often find myself having to stop something I might have started doing half way through, or have to rest a few times in between, because I get so tired and I feel so drained. It's as if someone has just pulled the plug out of your battery charger, you know what I mean [laughs]. And I've only got to sit down and shut my eyes, especially after lunch or of an evening, and I'm away.

Mr Taylor, meanwhile, put the matter in a more medical idiom:

> Well obviously, if you don't get the oxygen you haven't got the energy: you need oxygen to burn energy. So consequently, you tend to get very tired, very easily, and you feel very lethargic. You sit there planning all the things you can do. Yet once you get onto your feet, you very soon you realise that it's all pie in the sky.

Indeed, problems of breathlessness and a lack of energy were frequently spoken of synonymously. Sufferers sometimes had difficulty distinguishing one from the other. The other interesting theme in the accounts given above is that of the separation of mind and body – the classic *Cartesian dualism*. That is to say, respondents frequently tended to convey a sense of what may be termed 'bodily betrayal' (Goffman 1963) – a theme succinctly captured in another respondent's remark that 'the mind's willing but the body's weak'. Perhaps not surprisingly, this inability to translate one's thoughts, desires and wishes into bodily or somatic capacity tended to lead to considerable distress, frustration and depression.

Another important facet of the disease, of course, concerns the problematic character and nature of chronic coughing and sputum production. Quite apart from their social and symbolic significance, such symptoms tend to generate considerable distress and debilitation. As Fagerhaugh's (1975) earlier quote suggests, one of the main problems of chronic cough and sputum production is that it tends to trigger off acute respiratory distress. As Mr Kerr put it, concerning his chronic cough and sputum production:

> Oh it's with me practically all day long. Well up till you came just now, that's been six times this morning, that's how I go on all day long. And during the night, I've gotta get up, 'cause if I don't get up I can't breathe, I can't sleep, I can't do nothing. Oh it's a terrible business, it's an awful feeling when you're like that, well you can't explain it really. You've just gotta hang on the door up there till it eases itself. A few minutes, and after that it'll ease off a bit, you know, you can breathe a bit better then. But the first few minutes are horrible, absolute hell.

Later on in the interview in the course of discussing what he felt to be the major problem(s) he elaborated further:

> Well the way I am generally . . . the breathing, trying to get the sputum up, you know, a combination of things really. . . . Oh it's terrible that is [coughing and sputum production], it's terrible when that starts, you're hanging on the door, cough, cough, cough, and she's [wife] banging on me back tryin' to help fetch it up, oh it's terrible. Sometimes it takes a terrible long while to get it up, you're weakened right out, it drains and weakens you completely, very debilitating it is.

Also, the more general issue regarding the perennial problem of chest infections means that individuals have to be continually on their guard against the possibility of contracting one. At the first sign of an infection prompt action has to be taken in order to combat it. Indeed, in Williams' (1990) study, the military analogy or metaphor was often used in attempting to describe such vigilance. Terms such as 'guard against', 'vigilance', 'combat', 'battle', 'fight it' and 'kill it' were frequently used to describe the policy regarding chest infections. Such a response was understandable for, as one sufferer put it, 'if a chest infection strikes, it really tends to drag me down and weaken me out'. Thus vigilance, together with the continual monitoring of signs (such as the colour of the sputum) and symptoms of a potential chest infection, was of the utmost importance.

As mentioned in Chapter one, in addition to these 'main' symptoms of COAD, studies have also indicated that in certain more advanced cases, patients tend to develop blood gas abnormalities such as hypoxaemia (oxygen deficiency) and/or hypercapnia (excessive CO_2 retention). Consequently they tend to suffer from varying degrees of neuro-psychological impairment or deficit (Prigatano and Grant 1988). This tends to lead to certain cognitive and psychological problems of varying nature and severity, which include the following: diminished levels of alertness, confusion, obtundation, difficulty concentrating for very long, forgetfulness, headaches and in certain cases anxiety, irritability and restlessness. Thus in Williams' (1990) study, for example, the problems which were mentioned tended to vary both in nature and severity. Forgetfulness was one such problem. As Mr Charlton remarked: 'I'm terribly forgetful these days, and I used to have a very good memory', whilst for others, such as Mrs Prout, the problem was a loss of concentration:

If I concentrate on things for very long, I find that my concentration begins to wander after a time. I can't seem to concentrate for very long. I restore antique china, and I'm only able to do it for a couple of hours, and I don't do it every day now. Because, after a time, I can't think any more about what I'm supposed to do, I get it all wrong, and that's not like me, or it wasn't. And I hope my brain isn't getting addled, 'cause it isn't the brain I had. . . . If my brain dies, if that goes, I might as well be dead.

A further complication of COAD is that, again in certain more advanced cases or stages of the disease, patients tend to develop right-sided heart failure (cor pulmonale) and other sequelae such as oedema of the legs and ankles. As discussed in Chapter three, the recommended form of treatment in such cases is oxygen therapy (often for up to 16 hours a day or continuously). Mrs White, for example, was one such case. She claimed that in addition to oedema of her legs and ankles, the swelling went right up to her stomach; something which she found considerably uncomfortable. Her legs felt 'permanently bruised', and when she really 'swelled up', she was unable to put her shoes on. She also claimed to have noticed that when she really 'swelled up', her breathing became much worse and that, besides the swelling being generally uncomfortable and a nuisance, it was also quite painful. Consequently she had been put on diuretics in order to try to help reduce the swelling. Similarly Mr Thomas described his legs and ankles as being like 'two bleedin' barrage balloons'. Both were having oxygen therapy –

Mrs White virtually continuously and Mr Thomas for 16 hours a day – which, as Chapter three discusses, may cause further problems in sufferers' lives.

Psychological sequelae

As Dudley *et al.* (1980) note, a disease that interferes with breathing, reduces energy and vitality, and which produces progressively worsening, though fluctuating, symptoms, usually tends to produce psychosocial complications. Although not strictly speaking a direct symptom of COAD, feelings of anxiety, irritability, frustration and depression are frequently experienced by sufferers. Consequently, in sufferers' minds they may come to form as much a part of the experience of COAD as being breathless and suffering all the other associated symptoms discussed above. As a range of studies have shown, COAD patients often tend to become anxious, depressed and socially isolated (Dudley *et al.* 1980). Indeed, the prevalence of psychiatric illness in this disorder may be as high as 50 per cent (Rutter 1977), whilst a recent study by Rosser *et al.* (1983) reported that 60 per cent of their sample were potential 'cases' according to the General Health Questionnaire.

Research has also indicated a tendency for patients with COAD to become withdrawn, to avoid social interaction (Lester 1973), to be socially isolated, lonely and anxious (Lustig *et al.* 1972), and to rely on psychological coping mechanisms of 'isolation of affect, denial and repression' (Dudley *et al.* 1980). For example, Lustig and colleagues described COAD patients as 'highly anxious, socially isolated, lonely, and afraid to commit themselves to vocational activities' (1972: 322). Dudley *et al.* (1973) observed that many severely disabled COAD patients tend to live in 'emotional strait jackets'; no longer able to become angry, depressed, or even happy, due to any significant emotional changes triggering distressing symptoms. Similarly, Lester (1973) found that COAD patients tend to opt for a constricted 'living space', both spatially and socially, involving a withdrawal into the home and avoidance of social interaction with others.

One of the commonest psychological states amongst COAD patients is that of depression (Dudley *et al.* 1980). For example, in McSweeny *et al.*'s (1982) study, of a total of 150 COAD patients assessed by the Minnesota Multiphasic Personality Inventory (MMPI), 42 per cent exhibited evidence of significant depression compared to a figure of 9 per cent amongst age-matched controls. There have also been some attempts to describe the personality of COAD patients utilising various instruments such as the MMPI. However, these findings must be interpreted with caution. Lester (1973), for example, found that patients scored significantly above 'standard levels' on the hypochondriasis, depression and hysteria (a triumvirate referred to as the 'neurotic triad') scales of the MMPI. However, as Grant and Heaton (1985) point out, many different groups of chronically ill patients also exhibit significant elevations of these scales and hence such elevations are not COAD-specific. Also, Logan and Johnson (1974) reported significant elevations in COAD patients of the 'psychopathic deviance' (covering, amongst other things, a resistance to close personal ties) and 'psychasthenia' (which includes worry and anxiety) scales. However, as Dudley *et al.* note: 'these elevated scores may be related to an understandable response to dyspnoea' (1980: 415). Thus it is questionable whether such elevations are specific to COAD patients. Indeed, Dudley *et al.* (1980) did not detect elevations on these scales in their predominantly upper-middle-class group of COAD patients, compared with the predominantly lower economic class samples of Lester (1973) and Logan and Johnson (1974). As Dudley *et al.* note, this may suggest a 'positive relationship between social class and adjustment to the disease process' (1980: 415). Studies have also shown that older COAD patients tend to report fewer emotional problems, including depression, anger and frustration, than their younger counterparts (Guyatt *et al.* 1987). This finding is consistent with a study by Cassileth and colleagues (1984), which found lower levels of depression and anxiety in older patients across a broad range of chronic illness conditions.

In Williams' (1990) study, frustration and depression owing to the limitations imposed by the illness, and the time taken to accomplish simple, hitherto taken-for-granted daily tasks, were also commonly experienced problems. Whilst 7 per cent stated that they never or only rarely experienced frustration, 38 per cent admitted to sometimes feeling this way, and 55 per cent confessed that they often experienced frustration due to the limitations which the illness imposed upon them. The figures for depression were 33 per cent, 27 per cent and 40 per cent respectively. It was also found that women tended to score higher than men in terms of general psychological distress: a finding which is in line with other studies which generally tend to report higher rates of psychiatric disorder amongst women than men (Goldberg and Huxley 1980). Furthermore, as in Guyatt *et al.*'s (1987) and Cassileth *et al.*'s (1984) studies, although the relationship was relatively weak, older people tended to report fewer emotional and psychological problems, such as frustration and depression, than their younger counterparts. Thus, accounts such as the

following were fairly typical of the frustration and depression which
sufferers in Williams' (1990) study experienced as a consequence of
COAD. First, Mrs McLeod:

> It's very frustrating. Really all I do is just sit about these days, reading
> or doing crosswords, watchin' a bit of telly, you know. I mean, I see
> jobs around the house that need doing and I can't do them any more,
> and I get very frustrated and upset about it at times.

And concerning depression she stated:

> Sometimes, especially when I'm left in here on me own, I get to
> thinking: 'I don't know what I'm living for', 'not worth living like
> this', you know, more or less feeling sorry for meself I suppose
> [laughs].

Mr Brown, meanwhile, painted a very stark, bleak, picture:

> I'll tell you, sometimes I feel, when you're in the middle of an attack,
> I feel as though, wouldn't it be easier to throw meself off over the
> flippin' balcony! Now I've never felt anything like that in my life
> before, but at times that's how you feel. When you can see no light at
> the end of the tunnel, of course it makes you think things that normally
> you would never dream of doing. . . . There isn't a man alive who's
> had to go through this sort of thing without getting a feeling of
> frustration and depression.

Others, however, such as Mr King, appeared somewhat more
philosophical:

> Well at times I do get frustrated, because I'm so restricted in
> everything I do. Everything takes so much longer to do, and there are
> so many things I can't do any more, I'm very restricted nowadays. But,
> well, you just have to learn to accept it, accept the limitations. There
> are plenty of people worse off than myself. 'Cause if you don't try and
> come to terms with it, accept it and learn to live with the limitations,
> well you'd probably drive yourself crazy.
>   I've also been fortunate in that I've not really suffered from severe
> depression over this thing. Sure you get your down days when things
> seem worse than usual. But when you're disabled like I am, you've got
> time to reflect on everything and you realise that there are many ways
> of viewing the same situation. You know, a glass can be half empty or
> half full, depending on your point of view. So I try and be
> philosophical about these things, you know, you can always think of

others who are worse off than yourself can't you? I figure that if you look at it any other way, well you'd end up a very bitter, miserable man.

Yet despite the fact that frustration and depression are commonly experienced in relation to COAD, sufferers' accounts often conveyed the sense of struggle which most were engaged in: namely, one of trying not to let such feelings get a hold or a grip of them, and hence drag them down still further. In short, the struggle with, or battle against, a chronic illness takes place not only within the bio-physical realm, but also on the psychological and social terrain. Moreover, the following quotation from Mr Brown highlights the altogether quite different nature of the problems which a chronic, *vis-à-vis* short-term acute, illness poses for the sufferer. Essentially, as he put it, this concerns the fact that '. . . my illness is with me all the time, twenty-four hours a day, day in, day out'. Such problems do not simply go away with the passage of time. Rather, if anything, regarding COAD symptoms at least, they become progressively worse.

SYMPTOM VARIABILITY AND THE ROLE OF 'TRIGGERS'

An essential aspect of the experience both of COAD in general and dyspnoea in particular concerns its quite variable nature and the manner in which it may be 'triggered' by other endogenous and exogenous factors. Indeed, many in Williams' (1990) study found this one of the most perplexing aspects of their condition. Mr Ash, for example, echoed the sentiments of many patients when he said: 'We just have to take it day-by-day, 'cause you never can tell what you're going to be like tomorrow, no two days are alike. See today I'm pretty good, whereas tomorrow I might not be very good at all.' Not only do symptoms vary from day to day, they also vary diurnally. Mr King, for instance, spoke of how his symptoms were very much worse first thing in the morning, and offered his own quasi-medical explanation as to why:

I'm also much much worse in the mornings. I have a real job getting going in the mornings. The evenings aren't so bad, because I've been on my feet and using my lungs during the day you see. But I suppose that when you've been lying in bed all night – well actually I have to have pillows to prop me up – you're not using the lungs so much, they've not been fully operational like they are during the daytime, and so that's probably what causes the problem in the mornings. It's very, very hard for me to get up in the mornings. I mean, just getting out of bed makes me breathless and I have to sit on the edge of the bed until it passes.

Moreover, not only are sufferers faced with diurnal and day-to-day variations in their symptoms, they also have to contend with various other external triggers such as the weather and climatic conditions; things which contribute considerably to such symptom variability. Thus, COAD sufferers are forced to become 'lay meteorologists', having to pay careful attention to (fluctuating) climatic conditions. As Mr King remarked:

Oh . . . the weather makes an awful difference. If it's humid, you're in terrible, terrible trouble, because there's no air you see, you just don't have the air. And I notice it's the same when it's damp. When you go out and it's damp it's absolute murder to walk in. Then of course there's the cold weather, the cold weather wipes you out completely. In other words if it's too hot or too cold, if it's humid or it's damp, you're in trouble. If it's in between, a day like today for instance, then it's not too bad, because there's fairly good air and, umh, you can breathe pretty well then. Weather like this helps quite a lot you see . . .
Then of course there's windy weather, I just can't make it in windy weather at all. I have great difficulty breathing if I happen to go against it. . . . So I have to avoid going out in windy weather as it increases the breathing problems no end. And of course, you just can't walk into a strong head wind with this condition anyway, because you'd begin to over-exert yourself and you'd become very short of breath. . . . Also, if there's any kind of smoke, fumes or smog about when you're out, especially exhaust fumes from the cars and buses and what have you, then it's murder to breathe. And if you're anywhere where there's smoking then you're in real trouble. So you have to try and avoid all these things, this is what you're up against all the time.

A further important aspect of the experience of COAD concerns the manner in which dyspnoea is susceptible to being 'triggered' by anxiety, general psychological distress or (over-)emotional involvement of any kind. Thus, social situations which are 'anxiety provoking' tend to trigger off acute exacerbations of dyspnoea. This in turn tends to lead to further anxiety, thus resulting in both a crippling and a highly distressing vicious circle which can be difficult to break out of (Dudley *et al.* 1969, 1980). As Dudley *et al.* state:

Psychological states of action, such as a significant degree of anxiety, anger, and euphoria, are associated with increased energy expenditure, elevated ventilation, high oxygen consumption and skeletal muscle tension; while psychological states of non-action, such as apathy, depression, and deep relaxation, are associated with reduced energy expenditure, decreased ventilation, low oxygen consumption, and skeletal muscle relaxation. Either of these extreme states may increase symptoms in the [COAD] patient.

The dyspnoea produced by states of extreme action or non-action tends to increase the patient's psychological reactions which, in turn, produce more physiologic change. This physiologic change typically increases the dyspnoea, completing a vicious circle which may completely incapacitate even level I or II patients whose pulmonary function is relatively intact.

(1980: 416)

Many of those in Williams' (1990) study alluded to this 'vicious circle' effect, which often led to sufferers avoiding 'anxiety provoking' situations and withdrawing from social interactions with others. For example, Mr O'Riley said he had noticed that getting 'tense and panicky' when short of breath 'makes it worse. I've noticed that, you make yourself worse if you panic. So I try my hardest not to now.' Similarly, Mr Ash said that: 'If you get tense, if you get very tensed up, it seems to affect the breathing, it makes you even more breathless. It's a vicious circle really.' Mr Charlton, meanwhile, in a slightly different vein, stated:

> I'll tell you what I've noticed. If something's worrying me, if I've got something worrying me or gettin' me tensed up or nervous or something, then I seem to be breathless all day. If something's worrying me and I've got it on me mind, then I'm breathless all day.

SOCIO-PSYCHOLOGICAL MANAGEMENT STRATEGIES AND ISSUES OF SYMPTOM CONTROL

As Fagerhaugh (1975) suggests, COAD sufferers are constantly having to make strategic decisions concerning the selective allocation of their limited resources; what she terms basic mobility resources (BMRs: e.g. physical, temporal, social, economic and material). A diminished lung capacity, resulting in both a reduced oxygen supply and a reduced energy reserve, together with the frequently distressing and frightening consequences of getting out of one's 'depth', means that COAD sufferers face considerably difficult strategic management decisions regarding the selective allocation of their BMRs. Patients must allocate their limited lung capacity and energy reserves both carefully and strategically to the tasks they must do, or wish to do. Hence, 'two key issues for them are symptom control (energy loss) and the balancing of regimen versus other considerations' (Fagerhaugh 1975: 99). In particular, tasks and activities constantly have to be 'gauged' in terms of both their 'oxygen cost' and their energy consumption (Fagerhaugh 1975). Consequently, some tasks and activities have to be dropped or cut out, whilst other more essential ones have to be approached and negotiated in a different manner in order to avoid further symptomatic distress. Moreover, as we shall see in Chapter four, the ability to perform even basic tasks and activities such as walking and talking is considerably reduced. It is in such contexts that COAD sufferers are continually having to 're-normalise' (Weiner 1975) their expectations in line with their increasing incapacity and decreasing resources.

Many of those in Williams' (1990) study, for example, spoke of the basic management strategies which they adopted in order not to provoke or further exacerbate their symptoms. In this context, the 'pacing' of tasks and activities was often referred to: that is to say, adjusting tasks and activities to a pace which they found manageable without too much distress. Others spoke of how they broke or 'chopped' tasks up into smaller, more manageable components, or of how they did tasks one at a time now instead of simultaneously, resting in between – what one woman referred to as doing things in 'relays'. Many also highlighted the precarious balance which needed to be struck and the struggle this involved, between, on the one hand, maintaining as normal a life as possible given one's limitations (what Weiner [1975] terms 'keeping-up') and, on the other, stagnating, doing nothing and vegetating in the face of their symptoms (what Weiner [1975] terms 'giving-in'). COAD sufferers are constantly having to reconcile, juggle and balance the limitations and restrictions created by their reduced oxygen supply and other symptoms with the desire to remain mobile and maintain as normal a life as possible; what may be termed an attempt to 'hold on to normality'. Thus, respondents often spoke of attempting to 'remain as active as possible given the limitations and restrictions' of 'not giving in easily'; of 'getting there in the end'; of 'doing as much as I can for myself'; and finally of 'not letting others do, what I can do for myself, even if it takes me that much longer'. However, many were also fearful of 'doing too much' and 'getting out of my depth'. As Mr Brown suggested, this placed some in a 'catch twenty-two' situation as 'everything I attempt to do leaves me so breathless and distressed that I feel inclined not to do anything', leading in some cases to what others have termed an 'unrealistic fear of activity and dyspnoea' (Agle *et al.*

1973). This highlights the often considerable tension which exists between, on the one hand, a strategy of maximising activity and attempting to 'keep-up' and yet, on the other hand, a concern with the mimimisation and control of distressing symptoms (i.e. a battle between the social and the bio-physical imperatives). Moreover, as we shall see in Chapter six, another common response to the distressing symptoms of COAD concerns the tendency for sufferers to 'live in emotional strait jackets' and withdraw from social interaction (Dudley *et al.* 1973, Lester 1973).

All such strategies and attempts to devise such strategies are, of course, closely linked to the perceived sense of control which individuals feel they have over the illness and its symptoms. This is all the more important in the light of research findings which suggest that psychosocial factors play a contributory role in the degree of dyspnoea experienced even in the presence of severe lung disease (Rosser and Guz 1981, Jones 1988). For example, Burns and Howell (1969) found that COAD patients who were 'disproportionately breathless' exhibited higher rates of emotional distress than the remainder of COAD patients within their study. Furthermore, their dyspnoea improved with the resolution of these emotional disturbances. Similarly, in Williams' study (1990, Williams and Bury 1989a, b), only moderate correlations (0.38 (p <.001)) were found to exist between lung function (FEV_1 percentage of predicted values for age, sex and height) and dyspnoea (oxygen-cost diagram). Whilst in contrast, a higher correlation (-0.68 (p <.001)) was found to exist between ratings of general psychological distress (General Health Questionnaire -12) and dyspnoea (oxygen-cost diagram). As Mrs Prout put it:

> sometimes I get out of breath . . . and I have to do peak flow counts and these are *very high.* And yet sometimes I'm gasping for breath, and I don't understand that.

Moreover, the ratings and accounts given by those in Williams' (1990) study regarding their perceived degree of control over the illness varied considerably, and fairly independently of the degree of underlying physiological impairment. Thus there were some who felt that they had a 'fair' or 'moderate' degree of control over their illness. Those who fell into these categories frequently spoke of how they knew exactly what to do in the event of a bad attack; of how they tried to remain calm and not panic when breathless; of how they adopted the correct breathing techniques ('the tricks of the trade' as one respondent called them); of how they knew exactly which situations they should not get into; and, finally, of how, with the aid of their medical regimens, they felt they managed to 'control it pretty well'. In contrast, others spoke of having 'no' or only a 'minimum' degree of control over their illness nowadays. Such respondents spoke of not feeling able to control their breathing any longer; of being frightened, panicking and feeling helpless in the event of a bad attack; and, more generally, of how the illness was bigger than they were these days as, 'everything I try to do, it beats me, I'm scuppered. . . . I ain't got no control over it, not now'. A similar pattern emerged when considering instead the perceived degree of severity sufferers accorded their illness.

Indeed, further statistical analysis of these data revealed some interesting differences between those having relatively poor lung function but who were less breathless, and those who had relatively good lung function but who were more breathless. In particular, the former group tended to score lower on the twelve-item General Health Questionnaire ($p < .001$); rated themselves more highly in terms of their perceived degree of control over their illness ($p < .05$); were less likely to get a feeling of fear and panic when short of breath ($p < .05$); rated their illness less severely ($p < .005$); and were less likely to accept that they were 'disabled' ($p < .005$). They also had a lower number of hospital admissions in the preceding year ($p < .01$); were more likely to be in full-time employment ($p < .05$); and, finally, were less likely to feel socially isolated ($p < .03$).

In summary, as other studies have indicated (Dudley *et al.* 1980, Jones 1988), it is clear that psychosocial factors, together with the coping and management strategies devised and adopted, play a significant role in the *experience* of COAD and its associated symptomatology, even in the presence of severe lung disease.

MEDICAL CRISES

As Strauss (1975) has noted, it is in situations such as those discussed above that issues concerning the occurrence and management of medical crises loom large. Patients and their families have to be prepared at all times – to be in a state of continual 'readiness' – for the occurrence and management of what may be a life-threatening medical crisis. Thus, as with all other aspects of their lives, sufferers' attempts to manage medical crises involve supporting kinsmen, particularly immediate family. For example, Mrs Brown, a respondent in Williams' (1990) study, whose husband suffered from COAD, described the occurrence of such crises in the following manner:

Oh sometimes, when he's had a sudden bad attack, he's passed out. It's happened a couple of times now. Once I had to telephone the hospital, 'cause I couldn't get his mouth open far enough to stop his tongue from going back into his throat and I panicked a bit. Oh it was frightening I'll tell you. . . . It's a terrible experience, and the worst thing is you never know when it's gonna happen. Well, when I have to go and do shopping and I have to leave him on his own, I worry about how he'll be when I get back, how I'll find him. So I hurry back, and as soon as I open the door I shout out: 'You all right Bill?', and if he says yes I breathe a sigh of relief; 'Thank God for that', you know. Oh it's a terrible worry, it's on your mind all the time, day and night, there's no escaping it. As I say, it's happened a few times. Once when we was out and fortunately there was a woman who was a nurse who helped us. But it also happens sometimes in the night and he's completely out, out to the world, he can be out for quite a time. Oh it's a terrible experience.

Similarly, Mr Kerr's wife had to be available at all times of the day and night – which sometimes involved having to be woken up twice a night – in order to help clear his chest, as an inability to get the sputum up tended to leave him 'very short of breath and frightened'. Mrs Bush, meanwhile, had been told by her doctor that if her husband became 'really bad', she should call an ambulance immediately rather than contact him. Unfortunately, this had happened fairly recently:

Mrs Bush: I thought that was it, I thought he was gonna die, 'cause he was that bad I had to call an ambulance. And I mean I cried as they took him out of the flat that morning.

Mr Bush: Yes it was so sudden see, no warning or nothing. I just couldn't get me breath, not even when I'd been on the nebuliser. Well then I did panic and I told the wife to call an ambulance. I mean I'd have to be bad before I'd do that, I don't cry wolf easy. It was very frightening, like a heart attack it was.

In short, the (ever present) possibility of medical crises adds a further potentially threatening dimension to the experience of attempting to live with and adjust to a chronic illness condition such as COAD. Sufferers and their families have to be in a continual state of readiness concerning the possibility of a medical crisis. As with the cardiac patient, this is particularly true of COAD as, in the event of a 'bad attack', by their very nature, COAD's symptoms tend to be perceived, however correctly or incorrectly, in just such life-threatening terms.

CERTAIN AND UNCERTAIN ILLNESS TRAJECTORIES

For some diseases the trajectories are fairly predictable. Their phases can be anticipated, and even the relative rate at which the phases will change. For other diseases – like multiple sclerosis – both the phases and their rates are quite uncertain. Of course, for any given person who is ill, the sequential phases may be fairly predictable, but when they will appear and disappear can be most uncertain. This matter of certainty and uncertainty is of utmost importance because the efficacy of social arrangements is so closely linked with the predictability of the trajectories. Uncertain trajectories help to maximize personal and familial hardships.

(Strauss 1975: 47)

This quote from Strauss succinctly summarises one of the key aspects in the experience of illness: namely, the degree of certainty or uncertainty surrounding the illness trajectory. As we have seen, COAD varies considerably on a day-to-day basis. Yet it also varies in terms of the nature, pattern and course of its general development over the years. Thus issues of uncertainty concerning both present circumstances and future prospects abound, adding a further cognitive and practical twist to the already considerable hardship COAD sufferers and their families face. Indeed, this was a commonly experienced problem for those within Williams' (1990) study. Mrs Cole, for instance, found the future course and development of her illness highly problematic and uncertain. All she had to go on was the experience of her own father who had had emphysema: 'well you don't know whether it's going to get any worse, I hope not. But I mean all I've got to go on is me father, I mean he was terrible.' Consequently, she was left to: 'Just hope it don't get any worse.' Mr King, meanwhile, described the issue of uncertainty, together with the difficulties he faced in planning ahead, in the following manner:

Planning's impossible, you just have to take it day-by-day. It's no good trying to plan ahead ... with this thing. ... The future's very, very problematic and uncertain for me. I just have to take it one day at a time.

Concerning the specific character and nature of the illness trajectory experienced in COAD, Mr Brown put the matter graphically, both literally and metaphorically, when he stated:

Well it's gradually got worse and worse over time. The resistance of my body is gradually being worn down over time by the disease. It's gradually destroyed my lungs, eaten away at them like a cancer . . .

How can I put it? It goes in stops and starts. If you had a graph and made a chart of it, you could see a sort of trend of gradual deterioration over time and then like, Wallop, it would sort of dip down and then flatten out for a while. It's when you have a bad turn or a chest infection, that's when you really go downhill.

Similarly, Mr Ash stated:

It's a slow progress with quick periods in between. It'll go on for years and then all of a sudden you'll go down a stage, you'll get a bit worse, you'll find out that you can't do something that previously you could have done. Then you'll go for a long period at that stage. Then you'll go down another stage and that's how you carry on, you know.

Mr Thompson, meanwhile, stated:

Well I think emphysema grinds its way sort of remorselessly on and, ah, you realise there's no significant landmarks as such. . . . The breathlessness has progressively and relentlessly got worse over the years, you know. I mean there are peaks and troughs, but the general trend is downwards. Not only the breathlessness of course, but also my physical ability to do things that once I could manage to do, they're the benchmarks if you like. But it's all very slow, it's very slow, but none the less it's inevitable. I mean it's been happening over the last what, 15–20 years or so I suppose, it's a very slow process, so there's been no sudden great changes. It's only when you look back that you really realise the extent of it, that your expectations of what you can and can't do have had to undergo a drastic revision.

One of the most commonly voiced fears regarding the future was of drifting into total dependency. Thus Mrs Cole remarked: 'Well I mean my worst fear is to finish up like my father, that's what I'm thinking, he was terrible. Ending up totally bedfast and dependent on other people, that's my worst fear.' Others expressed a fear of worsening symptomatology and of death itself. Thus Mr King remarked:

Well I have to be realistic about it. Let's face it, it's not going to get any better or stabilise, it's going to get progressively worse and worse. Now it depends on how long it's going to take and when it happens . . . I've figured out you see, well it's going to get worse and, ah, maybe I'll be lucky enough to get a heart attack or something like that before I become totally disabled. I would loathe getting like that, because I don't think I could ever stand being bed-ridden or anything like that, I couldn't take it. I find it hard enough to take as it is, but this is the one thing that I dread. Because I've figured out that, umh, if the breathing gets so bad that I become immobilised totally, well then I'd rather that I wasn't breathing at all any more!

And Mrs McLeod stated:

> Well my worst fear is of getting any worse, 'cause if me breathing gets any worse, well it's bad enough now, but if it gets any worse it would be frightening. My worst fear is of slowly suffocating, dying gasping for breath when I'm alone here in the flat on me own, that's my worst fear.

Such accounts concerning the uncertainty and unpredictability of the illness trajectory, together with the feelings and fears expressed about COAD's future course and development, convey a fairly chilling and disturbing picture. Yet despite these disturbing accounts, there were still signs of sufferers and their families attempting to mobilise, cling to or maintain hope and an optimistic outlook, however tentatively, in the face of their adversity. Thus the hope of stability was a frequently voiced sentiment; the hope that things would not get any worse. As Mr O'Riley put it: 'there's the old sayin' "Just hope and pray", you know', whilst Mr Bush stated: 'I just keep hoping against hope that things will not get any worse than they already are, just keep hoping for the best.' As the following chapter discusses, some may look to medicine for a solution to their problems, in the shape of either a new drug, a medical breakthrough or a heart and lung transplant. Others, however, like Mrs Prout, may find solace in things such as the church:

> I get great pleasure from it [the church] and I believe it gives me something, something extra to cope. . . . I derive great strength from the spiritual part of it.

Thus many sufferers and their families, despite being placed in a situation of considerable uncertainty and ambiguity surrounding the future, still attempt to mobilise a semblance of hope in the face of their adversity: a precious, yet precarious, balancing of what others have referred to as the 'hope of remission and/or relief' as against the 'dread of progression' (Weiner 1975). It is situations such as these which create further tensions and dilemmas; issues which have to be faced up to and reconciled by both sufferers and their families. Such difficulties add a further dimension of disadvantage to the already frequently downward spiralling experience of COAD.

NEGOTIATING A SETTLEMENT: LIVING WITH A CHRONIC ILLNESS

This chapter has attempted to convey something of the reality and experience of COAD and its associated symptomatology. Yet the foregoing discussion, together with the subsequent chapters, also illustrates something of the ingenuity and tenacity of many COAD sufferers and their families in the face of their adversity; of the positive as well as the negative aspects of their lives and styles of adjustment. Learning to live with a chronic disease engenders an appreciation of what others take for granted. Small, hitherto seemingly unimportant, things suddenly become significant. Mundane tasks and activities which are successfully accomplished become great achievements for the chronically ill, something from which a sense of personal satisfaction, accomplishment and independence may flow. By the limiting of expectations and aspirations, a small sense of contentment, satisfaction or even happiness may be gleaned from what others take for granted. In this respect Burton (1975) quotes the following passage from Solzhenitsyn's classic novel *A Day in the Life of Ivan Denisovich*:

> Shukov went to sleep fully content. He'd had many strokes of luck that day: they hadn't put him in the cells; they hadn't sent the team to the settlement; he got a bowl of kasha for dinner; the team leader had fixed the rates well, he'd built a wall and enjoyed doing it; he'd smuggled that bit of hacksaw blade through; he'd earned something from Tsezar in the evening; he bought that tobacco. And he hadn't fallen ill. He'd got over it. A day without a dark cloud. Almost a happy day.
>
> (Solzhenitsyn 1968: 142–3)

Thus, by learning not to take things for granted, by gaining pleasure from the seemingly small, insignificant things in life, by taking each day as it comes, and by mobilising at least a semblance of hope and optimism in the face of adversity, COAD sufferers may similarly manage to get through their days. Perhaps, one might say, not so much days without a dark cloud as days with patches of blue sky in between.

Chapter 3

Medical care

The lives of those suffering chronic illness conditions are inextricably linked with, and influenced by, medicine. Indeed, despite moves towards alternative forms of healing and the growth of self-help groups, orthodox medicine remains a key resource in the management of (chronic) disease. As Locker states:

> Doctors are usually the first experts that are consulted in the course of the illness career. They provide the clinical labels by which persons become officially chronically sick and signal the beginning of the process by which the disabled become segregated from society. . . . They provide the cognitive resources which help reduce pain and functional limitation, they are called upon to verify the disabled person's claims for benefits and services, and they have a significant impact on the illness career by influencing conceptions of self and defining appropriate conduct for the person concerned. Consequently medical decision making is of some importance in the social processes which lead to the development of disability and handicap. . . . Some have argued that the influence of medicine has extended beyond clinical concerns to the point where it now dominates the administration of services and benefits for chronically sick and disabled people, an involvement which does not always operate in the best interests of the recipients.
>
> (1983: 43)

As Locker's quote suggests, medicine can be both an *enabling* institution, one which solves or mitigates many problems, and yet, at one and the same time, a *constraining* one which may create or exacerbate other problems. Thus medical regimens, therapeutic interventions and all other aspects of the medical care process, whilst conferring great benefits, may also create their own problems and difficulties.

Yet the exact starting point of the chronically sick and disabled person's contact with and experience of medical care crucially depends upon the issue of illness behaviour in the face of early signs and symptoms of disease, together with the decision-making processes of *when* and *where* to seek medical help. These are particularly pertinent issues when considering COAD.

ILLNESS BEHAVIOUR AND THE DECISION TO SEEK MEDICAL HELP

As discussed in Chapter one, it is now widely accepted that COAD begins at a relatively early stage in life and is characterised by a slowly progressive, insidious, deterioration of lung function for many years prior to the development and presentation of frank clinical illness (Burrows 1985). Moreover, the perception of COAD on the patient's part is obviously subject to various psychosocial and cultural determinants, such that onset rarely coincides with the subjective perception and presentation of frank clinical symptoms. However, it remains possible that COAD can have a fairly abrupt onset, with a rapid decrease in ventilatory capacity occurring during the few years prior to the onset of symptoms (Burrows 1985). As Barstow notes:

The manifestations of pulmonary emphysema typically occur during the productive years of life. *Its course usually has become largely irreversible by the time the symptoms are fully evident.* The person gradually becomes aware that his energy level and ability to perform accustomed work has decreased in comparison to what is still able to be performed by his peers. His 'cigarette cough' has worsened and the amount of sputum he raises has increased; he may wheeze or 'pant' under stress or exertion. *Some of those afflicted with the condition may be unaware of the underlying pathologic process until an acute attack of dyspnea or pneumonia intervenes.*

(1974: 137; my emphasis)

The predominant pattern of illness behaviour and medical consultation in Williams' (1990) study of COAD out-patients, for example, was one of *delay*. That is to say, there tended to be a delay, often for a considerable period of time, between initial illness onset and subsequent medical consulation. Mr Wilkinson, for instance, was a good example of this predominant pattern of delayed medical consultation. He dated initial onset as being approximately ten or twelve years ago, and a considerable period of time seemed to have elapsed before he finally consulted his doctor. At one time 'a forty-a-day man', he explained:

I didn't go [to his GP], because I always put it down to just me smoking. I didn't go to the GP, not to that extent, only if I'd got something, you know, wrong with me. But I'd get a bit out of breath and, you know, as I say, I just put it down to smoking like.

Zola (1973), in his classic study of illness behaviour, found that most people tended to tolerate symptoms of illness for quite some time before finally going to the doctor. Furthermore, he found that the symptoms in and of themselves were not sufficient in explaining consultation. He identified the following five 'triggers' to consultation: the occurrence of an interpersonal crisis, perceived interference with social or personal relations, 'sanctioning' (i.e. pressure to consult by others), perceived interference with vocational or physical activity and, finally, 'temporalising of symptomatology' involving the setting of a deadline (e.g. 'If I feel the same way on Monday . . .').

The most frequently mentioned 'trigger' in Williams' (1990) study was the one concerning perceived interference with vocational or physical activity. It helped explain both delayed help-seeking and the *raison d'être* for finally consulting. Mr Bush, for example, a painter and decorator by trade, left it several years after initial onset before consulting his GP. At that time he did not regard his symptoms as serious, or at least as anything more than 'normal illness' (cf. Cornwell 1984), and relied on his own 'self-prescribed medications', resolving to take more care of his general health in future. It was only when his breathlessness began to become more troublesome and *interfere with his daily life* that he consulted his GP. He was then referred to hospital, diagnosed as having 'acute bronchitis', told that he should stop smoking and take care of his general health, and was prescribed a course of antibiotics, 'that was all at the time'. He gradually managed to 'wean' himself off smoking over the course of the next few years and did not bother to consult again until approximately four years later, when his breathlessness really became troublesome and began to *interfere considerably with his work*. It was only then that it became clear to him that he would have to see the doctor again as 'it was getting towards the frightening stage by then'. As he put it, up until this time he had been 'hoping that me condition would improve, praying that it would go away'. He then went back to his GP and was subsequently re-referred to the hospital, where he was given 'lots of tests' and was diagnosed this time as having 'emphysema'. Other reasons for delayed consultation included things such as the fear of diagnosis and subsequent hospitalisation, the lay advice of others (Freidson 1970) and the influence of economic considerations and constraints. As one respondent put it concerning the latter issue: 'in my mind if you didn't work you couldn't live, it was as simple as that. Looking back now I suppose I was pushing meself too hard.'

Unfortunately, an all too frequent consequence of the factors and processes described above is that the presentation and/or referral of COAD patients to specialist pulmonary care tends to occur late on in their illness careers when major, irreversible, damage to the airways and respiratory system has already been done and little can be done to help them.

The acquisition of a diagnosis

A considerable body of work now exists regarding the acquisition and impact of diagnosis (Anderson and Bury 1988, Robinson 1988, Scambler 1989). In particular, such work has highlighted the considerable uncertainty surrounding the pre-diagnostic phase of the illness, together with the positive and negative aspects of diagnosis. It is also the case that with many of the conditions hitherto studied, the dating of diagnosis can be specified in fairly precise terms, often being portrayed as a major event or landmark in the individual's illness career. Moreover, much of this research has tended to focus upon serious, sometimes life-threatening and often considerably stigmatizing conditions such as cancer, multiple sclerosis, rheumatoid arthritis, epilepsy or AIDS: conditions which, when diagnosed, one would perhaps *a priori* expect to have a considerable impact upon both sufferers and their families. This, in many respects, provides a sharp contrast to the situation found in relation to COAD. That is to say, both the diagnosis of COAD and its impact on patients tend to differ quite considerably from those conditions mentioned above.

In Williams' (1990) study, for example, it seemed that, as with the slow and insidious nature of COAD's onset, the issue of diagnosis itself frequently could be characterised in a similar fashion. That is to say, patients often spoke of how the diagnosis had tended to shift over the years from something relatively benign such as 'a touch of bronchitis' or 'just a chest infection', to something altogether more severe in nature such as 'chronic obstructive bronchitis', 'emphysema' or finally, in a few cases, a 'closing of the airways' or even 'chronic obstructive airways disease' (for the reasons discussed in Chapter one, only a few in the study were chronic asthmatics). The case of Mr Bush, for example, showed clearly how the diagnosis had shifted from initially a relatively benign one of 'acute bronchitis' to the more threatening one of 'emphysema'. In short, whilst the reality of the disease was never in question, diagnosis, as portrayed by those in Williams' (1990) study, often appeared to be a rather hazy and vague affair which was difficult to pin-point exactly. Hence, in contrast to certain other chronic conditions and in line with the clinical nature of COAD as such, the concept of a 'creeping' or 'insidious diagnosis' seemed more appropriate.

Partly as a consequence of this 'creeping diagnosis', there was also a tendency for the impact of the diagnosis as such to be fairly negligible. After all, a moment's pause for reflection will confirm that to be told you have 'a touch of bronchitis', 'a bit of chest trouble' or even later on 'emphysema' or 'COAD' is a very different thing to being told that you have, say, cancer: the difference between what most laymen, however correctly or incorrectly, would regard as a relatively benign or 'normal' illness *vis-à-vis* a far more 'serious', life-threatening or terminal one. This is not to suggest that there were no cases in which the revelation of the diagnosis had a substantial impact upon the patient concerned; indeed there were, but they tended to be in the minority. More often, however, when a diagnosis was conferred it tended to be greeted in a matter-of-fact sort of manner, or, particularly concerning the revelation of 'emphysema' or 'COAD', without any real prior knowledge or understanding of what exactly these terms meant. For example, Mr Thompson's comments on his reaction to his diagnosis were instructive:

> Well I suppose really, I mean I'd known there was something wrong, that there was some problem and that it wasn't right, and I knew what my father was like, so it didn't come as a great shock to me. It's a sort of family problem really of chest complaints, so it wasn't a terrible shock to me.

In contrast, Mrs McLeod claimed she had no prior knowledge of emphysema and consequently was unclear what exactly it was when diagnosed as having it:

> Well I didn't know what it was at first, until the doctor told me, he explained to me, he told me I had emphysema. And I said to him: 'What's that?' 'Well,' he said, 'it's pretty bad, your lungs are like elastic sponges and yours are over-stretched. You've lost the natural elasticity of your lungs. Therefore they don't go in and out and so you're not getting half the air you should'. . . . He just said that that was it sort of thing, and that there was nothing they could really do about it, it was incurable. . . . Well I was a bit shocked at first, but I've just had to accept it sort of thing.

Yet as other studies have similarly found, it is none the less the case that the conferral of a diagnosis, however serious, may be greeted with a certain amount of relief, signalling as it does, the end of a period of considerable uncertainty and worry. Thus in Mr King's case, for instance, the acquisition of a diagnosis was in many respects greeted with a sense of relief, ending a period of quite considerable uncertainty on his part. As he put it, concerning both the pre-diagnostic phase and his feeling surrounding the acquisition of a diagnosis:

Mr King: Well naturally I was worried, all sorts of things go through your mind when you haven't been told what it is, you worry an awful lot. You begin to wonder what is wrong, you know, what is wrong? . . . So naturally I felt very worried until I finally found out exactly what it was.

Interviewer: How did you greet the diagnosis of emphysema?

Mr King: Well really I didn't know what it was, I'd heard of it, but I had no real idea what it was. I had to get a medical dictionary and look it up and see what it was. And I read that it was a distention of the lungs and what have you, and I tried to learn as much as I could about it. . . . But you see, the worst thing is not knowing, not knowing exactly what it is. Once you're told, once they've actually given you the diagnosis and you've found out a little bit about what you've got, exactly what the disease is, then at least you're in a better position to start to try and come to terms with it. You see you've got no other choice really. . . . It's when you don't know, when you haven't been told, that's the worst part, you tend to worry.

These accounts serve to convey something of the range of experience regarding illness behaviour and the acquisition of a diagnosis in relation to COAD. However, it is to the end result towards which such processes lead that this chapter now turns; namely, the experience of medical care.

PROBLEMATIC ASPECTS OF MEDICAL CARE IN COAD

Respiratory function tests and assessment procedures

An important aspect of the care and management of COAD, of course, concerns the regular monitoring of patients' respiratory functioning together with the assessment of their physical capabilities. Thus, in addition to various spirometric measures of lung function and the measurement of blood abnormalities, 12-, 6- or 2-minute walking distance tests (McGavin *et al.* 1976, 1978), cycle ergometry, paced stepping and treadmill exercises are frequently used in order to assess exercise tolerance and capacity. Yet, whilst from a medical viewpoint these provide essential information, from the point of view of the patient who dreads sustained exercise for any length of time, such tests, which are likely further to exacerbate their respiratory distress and anxiety, may appear unethical or punitive (Williams 1989b). In Williams' (1990) study, for example, some patients spoke of their fears and concerns regarding a trip to the respiratory function unit, or what another patient referred to as 'the chamber of horrors'. This was particularly so for patients who had had to struggle to get to their out-patient appointments via public transport – often involving a considerable expenditure of time, energy and money on their part – and hence wished to conserve their depleted energy reserves for the journey back home again. Miss Bell, for example, dreaded it whenever the doctor asked her to go to the respiratory function unit. As she put it:

> Oh I dread it, I really do, 'cause I don't do very well, I can tell . . . and I get all shaky, worked up and breathless. As soon as the doctor tells me I've gotta go down there I get all worried and tensed up. . . . Having to blow into that machine's a real effort and, I tell you, I'm really whacked out. And then I've got to negotiate the walk from the hospital back to the station. Honestly, by the time I get home I'm really tired, it really takes it out of you. I hate those tests.

Moreover, as discussed below, patients may understandably feel somewhat aggrieved if, having gone through such tests, the results are not reported back to them.

The communication of information

As many studies have shown, one of the main areas where patient dissatisfaction tends to occur concerns the communication of information (Fitzpatrick 1984); those suffering chronic illness being no exception. Indeed, as Locker states:

> It could be argued that the communication of information is even more important with respect to chronic illness since the patient not only has to manage a variety of distressing symptoms but also has to learn to adapt to new and more limited life styles. Some would go as far as to claim that for many chronic illnesses the communication of information is *the* only form of treatment there is.

> (1983: 53)

Thus in Williams' (1990) study, for example, whilst general levels of satisfaction with health care were high, just over 30 per cent were either in some way critical or had 'mixed feelings' about the information they had received about their condition, and felt in need of more information. Similarly, many of those in Nocon and Booth's (1991) study of asthma were dissatisfied with the information they had been given. In particular they wanted to know more about possible aetiological factors in asthma, the management of attacks, when to summon medical help, the nature of drugs and their side-effects, the likely prognosis, the practical implications of their condition, and where to obtain further advice, help and support.

Obviously there are many reasons for the information and communication problems which occur between doctors and patients. Blaxter (1976) discusses the role of the following: organisational failures, misunderstandings (or a failure to ask) on the part of patients, the therapeutic management of information, and, finally, genuine clinical uncertainty. It may also be due to the doctors' operational ideologies of patient management, together with their images of patients and the doctor–patient relationship from which decisions and rules about information-giving stem (Locker 1983).

Whilst it was not possible, with any degree of certainty, to discern from patients' accounts which of these reasons, or combinations of reasons, was responsible in any one particular case, a common theme of dissatisfaction in Williams' (1990) study concerned the lack of any detailed and specific discussion of the patient's own *particular* case. Thus Mr Thomas, for example, discussed the need for doctors to be more 'aggressive' in their information-giving practices. His account is worth quoting at length, as it highlights many of the themes underlying patients' dissatisfaction with the giving of information:

I mean, for a long time I was just told that it was bronchitis and that I should pack up smoking. It's only since I've been under the hospital in the last, what, 6 years or so, that I've managed to obtain any sort of *real* information about me condition. They diagnosed emphysema. But really, I mean I've just been given a word, that's all, no sort of real explanation or discussion about it from the doctors at all. I mean I really want to know more about this heart condition [cor pulmonale] they say I've got now, you know, the extent of the damage done like. All I know is that me lungs are damaged, and that through a lack of oxygen through me lungs me heart's damaged. But I don't know *how much damage* is done to it, *how serious* it is, *how badly damaged me lungs are, what me chances are.*

I remember having an ECG and asking the doctor about it. And he said to me: 'Your heart is OK Mr Thomas, it's fine. There is nothing wrong with your heart.' And I said: 'Oh that's good, that's nice to hear, at least that's all right.' Next thing I know they're sayin' me bleedin' heart's damaged! Honestly, you end up not knowing *who* or *what* to believe. Now that's what annoys you . . . I mean one day I was in there [hospital], and I overheard a couple of doctors talking . . . about 17 per cent lung capacity or something or other. I only found out later that they were talking about my lungs! Well why the hell didn't they turn round and say to me. This is what I say, they should tell you the truth, be that little bit more 'aggressive' with you basically. Why didn't they say to me: 'Look Mr Thomas, you're only working on 17 per cent of your actual 100 per cent lung capacity', and show me on the screen. And I was still working then. I still didn't think there was anything seriously wrong at that time. But I'd much rather they told me, told me the truth, told you straight, 'cause then you know what you're up against don't you.

A related source of dissatisfaction occurred when those who desired more information were not given the results of their tests. As Mr Brown stated:

> You never get the results of them [tests] do you. Nobody ever turns round and says: 'Well Mr Brown, your lung function is well below', you never find out anything like that. You go for all these tests, but you're never told the results. It makes you wonder what it's all for.

And Mr Thomas remarked:

> You're only told the results when you ask the doctors direct, and even then they'll mostly just pass a comment like 'A little better', 'No improvement' or 'Slightly worse'. . . . Take last week for instance . . . when I went in there [to see the doctor] I had the envelope open looking at it [the results of his respiratory function tests]. . . . Well I ain't gonna find out any other way am I?

A final source of conflict, or potential conflict, for a few patients within Williams' study concerned the issues of causation. That is to say, some were critical of the way in which some doctors emphasised the causal role of smoking *vis-à-vis* other factors in accounting for the genesis of their illness. For example, Mr Doyal was critical of the emphasis doctors placed upon smoking – 'Doctors always say: "Oh, your smoking", it sickens you' – believing instead that years of exposure to car fumes and pollution in the City whilst working as a window cleaner, coupled with his involvement in a fire, were primarily responsible for his condition. Indeed, most respondents, whether critical of the doctors' emphasis upon smoking or not, tended to operate with a *multi-causal* framework concerning the aetiology of their condition. Thus whilst 11 per cent rejected smoking as a causal factor and 12 per cent accepted it as the sole cause, the majority (77 per cent) believed that other factors such as dust, air pollution, contact with asbestos and noxious fumes at work, in addition to smoking – which could play either a predominant or a peripheral role – were of causal importance in the aetiology of their condition. Thus, when asked which factors had contributed to his condition, Mr Ash gave the following response:

Mr Ash: Well a lot of things really, a combination of many different things. Smoking, and I used to work in a boiler house.

Mrs Ash: And then you got burned up by that mustard gas, he was in the airforce.

Mr Ash: Oh yeah, mustard gas, I got burned by mustard gas years ago. So it was a combination of things really, every little bit helped. . . . So I think that [mustard gas] must have played its part. And then there was smoking and the fumes from the boiler, sulphur fumes, 'cause a long time ago I worked as a boiler mechanic you see. And I also came into contact with asbestos, there's a little bit of asbestos mixed in with it too I think. . . . And I mean generally there was a lack of information at the time, you know, 'bout the dangers of smoking and asbestos.

Mrs Ash: And his father died of emphysema, so it could be partly hereditary. Does it run in families?

The doctor–patient relationship

A further source of dissatisfaction may relate more directly to the nature and quality of the doctor–patient relationship as such. Thus, time spent in listening to, empathising with, understanding and supporting patients may be particularly valuable in the context of a chronic, disabling, illness. Mr Thomas, for example, was fairly critical of his GP for the following reasons:

I mean he's OK but he always seems to be in too much of a hurry. It's sort of: 'Yep, yep, yep' and before you know it you're out of the door, you know. At times I feel, I've felt like sayin' to him: 'Just sit there, shut up and listen to me', so that in the end I come away thinking; 'Yes he's heard me', you know.

Similarly, Mrs McLeod was critical of the doctor she used to be under at the hospital she attended:

I always felt with him, very nice man to talk to mind, but I always felt that he was 'passing you off'. It would be: 'Well, how are you?'; 'Oh, I'm not too bad thank you.' And then he'd say: 'Right, come and see me in six months', and that was it. And you'd have sat there for two hours and that was the attitude you got, you know.

Patients in Williams' (1990) study also expressed their dislike at having to see different doctors and being 'chopped and changed around'; preferring instead the chance to build up a one-to-one relationship with just one doctor over a period of time and the sense of continuity and mutual understanding this may foster. Mr Ash, for instance, found the change of doctors at the hospital out-patient clinic disruptive:

For about the first, say, two or three years, I was under, well I was seeing [Dr G] all the time and then, all of a sudden, in about a year, I found that I'd seen about four or five different doctors. And I found that a bit of a problem really, 'cause you've got no continuity at all. You've got to explain it all again really, start from scratch each time, and that can be very wearing. 'Cause you're out of breath to start with, and you get more and more out of breath trying to explain why you're out of breath [laughs]!

Another related source of tension or potential conflict in doctor–patient relations may, of course, arise when a different doctor or hospital prescribes medication, or facilitates the acquisition of aids or appliances, which are of benefit to the patient but which have not previously been tried or suggested. This tends to result in the patient feeling somewhat aggrieved at not having had them sooner. As Mrs McLeod stated:

When I think, all the time I'd been going to [Hospital X] and no-one had ever suggested giving me oxygen, whereas [Hospital Y] prescribed it for me . . . and they gave me a wheelchair too. And yet all the time I'd been going to [Hosptal X], no-one had ever said to me about oxygen, or wheelchairs or anything like that, you know.

A final source of tension or conflict in the doctor–patient relationship regarding COAD may, of course, occur when patients persist in smoking in the face of medical advice to the contrary. Most COAD patients who smoke claim they would like to stop, but often have little confidence in their ability to do so. In reviewing the literature on physician advice to stop smoking, Pederson (1982) found success rates of between 20 and 56 per cent for COAD patients, whilst others have found that between 66 per cent and 75 per cent of patients in respiratory rehabilitation programmes manage to stop smoking, often involving several attempts (Mausner 1970).

Whilst medical advice, encouragement and support may initially be forthcoming, ultimately, if smoking persists, despair or intolerance may creep in and the patient may be branded a 'waste of the doctor's time'. Yet, though an understandable reaction, the very real difficulties of attempting to stop what for many is a life-long habit and addiction, should not be lost sight of, and may not be just a matter of lacking will-power or of failing to heed rational medical advice. As McSweeny and Labuhn state:

> The reasons for [COAD] patients' particular difficulties in quitting smoking are complex. The insidious nature of the disease is one factor … patients are often not aware of the seriousness of their lung condition until the disease is fairly advanced. After diagnosis, the physician might not give strong enough messages about the need to quit smoking, or he might give inadequate information about quitting methods. Most patients are long-term heavy smokers. If they are addicted to nicotine, as is often the case, they have uncomfortable withdrawal symptoms … this may lead to emotional arousal and increased respiratory distress. Under these circumstances, it is not surprising that most patients are not successful in the initial attempts to quit smoking.
>
> Social factors also play an important role in patients' continued smoking. Cigarette smoking is an integral part of most patients' lifestyle. It is associated with many daily activities, and is used for various reasons including pleasure, tension reduction, relief of boredom and just habit.
>
> (1990: 405–6)

In the context of a chronic illness, time can often drag. Thus, for a long-standing smoker, reaching for a cigarette is perhaps an understandable, though not condonable, response to boredom, frustration and depression. Mr Wilkinson, for example, gave a good account of the difficulties he faced in giving up:

> I mean I've tried to give it up, it's not as if I haven't bothered, you

know. I've managed to cut it down to eight a day, but it's hard. blimmin' hard. I mean I know it's for me own good, but it's not bleedin' easy breakin' the habit of a life-time is it? Well I say a habit, you're addicted really aren't you? It's a drug isn't it, nicotine, it's a drug, not like heroin, but it's still a drug none the less and I s'pose I'm hooked.

What we see here is a strong concern to appear in the correct moral light and, perhaps more importantly with respect to chronic illness conditions, with appearing, or at least attempting, to co-operate and comply with 'rational' medical advice. Thus, as McSweeny and Labuhn suggest:

> Interventions need to address the biological aspects of smoking addiction (withdrawal symptoms) as well as psychosocial and lifestyle issues. Physicians will be more successful in their intervention efforts if they provide specific advice on how to quit and if they emphasize how smoking cessation can improve the patients' quality of life. Self-efficacy (confidence in one's ability to carry out recommended quitting strategies) is an important factor in quitting.
>
> (1990: 406)

Medical regimens and therapeutic intervention

Another highly important issue in the lives of the chronically sick and disabled, of course, concerns medical regimens. The medical treatment of these conditions varies according to the particular illness diagnosed, the consequent degree of impairment, symptomatology and the presence or absence of complicating factors amongst other things. However, regimens often include the judicial usage of antibiotics to treat infective exacerbations, techniques to clear the bronchi of excess secretions (such as postural drainage, vapour inhalations and mucolytic agents), physiotherapy, breathing exercises, beta-adrenergic agonists to obtain the maximum possible broncho-dilation (via aerosol or nebuliser), courses of oral corticosteroids and, in more advanced cases or in times of acute exacerbation, inhalation of oxygen (which may be for up to 16 hours a day or continuously). In addition, systematic respiratory rehabilitation programmes covering patient and family education, breathing (re-)training and graduated exercise, may also help COAD patients to learn how to cope with the debilitating and challenging effects of the condition as well as helping them to maximise 'function', both physically and psychosocially (Petty 1985, 1988).

Generally, of course, COAD patients derive a good deal of help and benefit from their medical regimens. In Williams' (1990) study, for example, the vast majority of patients expressed considerable gratitude for what the doctors had done, or tried to do, for them and, more specifically, regarding both the subjective and objective benefits their treatment and medical regimens afforded them. Thus, patients frequently referred to their inhalers as 'a real life line, they keep me mobile. I don't know what I'd do without them.' Similarly, for those who required them, nebulisers afforded even greater relief. As one patient put it: 'you can almost feel the airways sort of opening up again and you can breathe that much easier. Then, gradually, you begin to feel yourself calm down and relax again.' Oxygen therapy also conferred noticeable benefits for most of those who needed it, facilitating generally improved levels of energy and mobility tolerance, together with a reduction in the patients' subjective feelings of tiredness and lethargy. Similarly, most of those who were on corticosteroids, despite the risks of side-effects, noticed a considerable improvement in their breathing problems and, hence, were able to enjoy greater levels of exercise tolerance than would otherwise have been the case. As one patient put it: 'Well, when they first put me on them, after a couple of weeks, I was running around like a "normal" person and I thought I was cured.'

Yet despite the undeniable, and indeed welcome, gains and benefits which medical intervention and treatment regimens bestow, they may also create new problems and difficulties or exacerbate existing ones. As Strauss (1975) has suggested, medical regimens can be both *enabling* and *disabling* when placed in the context of sufferers' daily lives. Thus what, from a medical viewpoint, might seem beneficial to the patient may, from the patient's own perspective, impose 'unacceptable' demands and constraints upon an already highly compromised life style. Indeed, there are perhaps five key, though not necessarily complementary, dimensions or criteria in terms of which patients tend to evaluate their medical regimens. These are as follows: (1) the degree of *symptomatic or subjective relief* the treatment affords; (2) the extent to which it helps facilitate *independence in activities of daily living* (ADL); (3) the *risks and side-effects* involved; (4) the degree of *time, difficulty and restriction* it involves; and, finally, (5) the degree of *embarrassment or stigma* it evokes in self and others. Potential sources of conflict and tension in the doctor–patient relationship may occur owing to the doctor's predominant concern with the first three criteria *vis-à-vis* the patient's general concern with all these dimensions. Hence, with this conceptual framework in mind, it is to a more detailed discussion of certain problematic aspects of medical regimens, when viewed within the context of COAD patients' daily lives, that this chapter now turns.

(i) Nebulisers and oxygen therapy

Whilst the inhalation of a broncho-dilator may take only a few seconds or minutes out of one's day, the use of a nebuliser or oxygen consumes a considerably greater proportion of time. Being on a nebuliser can involve anything from intermittent usage, to use once, twice, three or four times a day for approximately 15 to 20 minutes on each occasion. Similarly, oxygen therapy can involve anything from intermittent or nocturnal usage, to usage from 8 to 16 hours a day or continuous usage day and night.

Patients in Williams' (1990) study were asked to rate the degree to which their medical regimen interfered with or restricted their life. Whilst 62 per cent rated it as interfering only 'minimally' or 'not at all', a sizeable proportion rated it as interfering either 'moderately' (19 per cent) or 'markedly' (20 per cent) with their daily lives and activities. As one may perhaps expect, those who fell into the latter two categories tended to be those on nebulisers and/or oxygen therapy. Indeed, even for those with 'portable' nebulisers, the fact that they regularly had to use them could be burdensome. Moreover, although relatively weak, this relationship appeared to be mediated by age: older patients using nebulisers and/or oxygen tended to rate their regimens as less of an interference and restriction to their lives than their younger counterparts. Others, however, emphasised the fact that they were so grateful for the relief the treatment accorded them that consequently they were not too worried about the drawbacks it posed in terms of their daily life. As Mr O'Riley remarked: 'I'm not really worried about that [interference and restriction of daily life] these days because it does me good. It's doing me a lot of good since I've started taking that [nebuliser].' In addition, some stressed the fact that, because of the illness, their lives were already restricted to such an extent that the additional rigours, demands and restrictions of the regimen mattered very little.

Some also expressed concern about becoming, or being, 'dependent' upon their regimens. Mr Bush, for example, claimed that he was now 'totally dependent' on his nebuliser. In particular he expressed considerable concern over the fact that he had now reached the stage where he was 'immobilised without it', and could no longer obtain any sustained sense of relief from inhalers. As he put it: 'when I'm still breathless, even when I've been on the machine, which is what happened last time I was admitted to hospital, that's when I begin to panic, 'cause there's nothing I can do then you see'. As Petty and Nett warn regarding oxygen therapy:

> Too much oxygen may be a problem, particularly when patients feel that if a little is good, a lot more will be better. This attitude can be dangerous as too much oxygen can sometimes reduce breathing, thus leading to a dangerous buildup of carbon dioxide [which] is potentially toxic.
>
> (1984: 63)

Thus Mr Kerr remarked:

> Oh I have it [oxygen], but I try to avoid it as much as I can, I don't want to get too addicted to it. But I've got to have it, couldn't go without it. . . . Well, my doctor [GP] said to me not to, he said: 'I know what it's like', but he said: 'Try not to keep having too much of it.' 'Cause apparently someone he sees went there, sitting there he said, and they didn't know how much of it they was taking. So he said to me: 'Only when you really need it.' But as I say, I've got to have it, I couldn't go without it.

Mrs Cole, meanwhile, who disliked her self-acknowledged dependence on oxygen, stated:

> You always feel, it's like you get to the stage where you're frightened to stay off it, if you know what I mean. At the set time you sort of think to yourself, 'Oh, I must go on it', you know.

Indeed, it was long-term oxygen therapy which tended to pose most of the problems and difficulties experienced by those in Williams' (1990) study. Mrs White, for example, was on continuous oxygen therapy. Despite the undeniable benefits this afforded her, she claimed that it was also a big additional problem, restriction and impediment to her leading or attempting to maintain anything approaching a 'normal' life style. As she explained, going out involved considerable planning on her part and a major logistic exercise which involved the crucial help of others:

> Oh yes, it [oxygen] is a big restriction, definitely. I mean to go out anywhere is a big problem, a right palaver, 'cause I can't go anywhere without it you see. For example, we went to Ramsgate last weekend to see some friends, and we had to take three cylinders with us for the day plus my nebuliser. And once we got there I couldn't go out anywhere, I had to stay in the flat. And I mean, we was supposed to go round to

see my step-daughter's new house. But I couldn't go, there was too much walking about involved, so I couldn't go with them. There's so much planning involved in going out anywhere, you can't just get up and do something spontaneously, on the spur of the moment like, it all has to be planned, organised and arranged in advance.

She also spoke of the considerable complexity of arrangements and the organisation involved in going visiting:

You see, if we see friends, then it's mainly at weekends, as my husband's around then and it's easier at the weekend. Because if I happen to go out during the week, then he's at work see. And so I have to arrange for the oxygen to be taken round the night before, so that it's there waiting for me when I get to wherever it is I'm going. So it's easier at the weekends when we can take it over with us in the car on the day. But I mean generally, as a rule, I try and go to my mum's on a Tuesday for the day, they only live five minutes down the road you see. And so one of me brothers will come round the night before, deliver the shopping and take the oxygen back to me mum's ready for Tuesday. So I mean, yes it is a restriction, not just for me but for me husband too really. I mean he can't go out of the house with me without having to lug great big oxygen cylinders about, you know. We can't just get in the car and go off like we used to be able to do, nothing's spontaneous any more, everything's got to be planned.

Moreover, as she explained, she also was limited in the amount of time she could spend outdoors by the capacity of her portable oxygen cylinder: a classic case of Goffman's (1963) concept of 'living life on a leash'. As she stated: 'I can only be out for as long as my portable oxygen cylinder lasts. I have to get back before that runs out. I mean I couldn't be without it.'

As Chapter six discusses in more detail, a common theme running through such accounts concerns what Kelleher (1988) terms the *loss of spontaneity*. That is to say, the previously taken-for-granted ability to do things on the 'spur of the moment' is, to a greater or lesser extent, a privilege which is denied the chronically sick and disabled. Hence, it can readily be appreciated how the additional rigours and demands which medical regimens may impose upon sufferers – particularly in the latter, more advanced stages of COAD – may significantly contribute to this loss of spontaneity; adding a further dimension of disadvantage to what are often already highly compromised lives.

The accounts given above serve to highlight what is for many an acute dilemma regarding medical regimens: namely, a struggle to balance the competing imperatives of, on the one hand, the minimisation of distressing symptoms via regimen adherence, and yet, on the other hand, trying to lead as 'normal' a life as possible given the limitations of the condition, and avoid becoming over-reliant, or wholly dependent, upon such medication.

(ii) Side-effects

A final problem regarding medical regimens concerns the issue of side-effects. Patients in Williams' (1990) study were asked if their medication produced any unpleasant side-effects: 22 per cent said that it did. These tended to be patients who were on (long-term) oral corticosteroid treatment, where reported side-effects included mood swings, weight gain, cataracts, stomach ulcers and osteoporosis. Mrs Prout, for example, a chronic asthmatic, had been on steroids for many years. As she explained, the doctors had twice tried, unsuccessfully, to take her off them, but: 'I was very very ill, very bad. I remember it vividly, it was the most frightening experience I've had, I was very bad. So they've kept me on them over the years, 'cause they help with the breathing an awful lot.' Unfortunately, however, she was, it seemed, paying the penalty in terms of the side-effects and complications she now experienced. As she stated:

> Well, I mean I don't know if these things are *directly* caused by the steroids, I mean some doctors tell me 'Yes' and others just shrug their shoulders. But I've got osteoporosis and that *is* a side-effect, I know that. . . . And I've had a lot of trouble with my stomach, peptic ulcers, and I've also had a lot of trouble with my kidneys in the last few years. . . . I have chronic back ache and pains in my legs. Well, I just take that to be osteoporosis . . . but it all seems to have developed since the steroid treatment.

Mrs Andrews, meanwhile, found weight gain a problem:

> Oh, the weight, that *is* terrible. I mean, I've never been big in my life. And I think them steroids, I wonder if that doesn't do more harm than good carrying all that weight about with me, you know, 'cause I've put on about two stone since I've been on them. . . . Oh it's terrible. I mean there's me face and all round here and me bust. Not on me arms or hands, no, but it seems that all the rest of me, me trunk and me head, that's where it's all gone to.

In contrast, Mr Bush had suffered from cataracts in both eyes; a well known side-effect of steroid treatment. In the latter stages he claimed that he had been left almost blind, and as a consequence had been practically housebound and unable to drive his car. At the time of interview he had recently had the cataract in his right eye removed, claiming that it had given him 'a tremendous lift', and was hoping to have the other one done in the very near future.

Finally, Mr Thompson described a somewhat different, more subtle and sinister change brought about when on steroids:

> When I'm on steroids they seem to affect my mood quite a bit. I seem to have tremendous energy, which I don't normally have, the adrenalin seems to flow quite readily and I'm quite alert. In fact I can't sleep, sometimes I don't sleep all night, I just can't seem to sleep when I'm on them, whereas normally of course, you're always ready to go to sleep. But after a fortnight of being on them, I then seem to go over the top. I can't describe it really other than a sort of nervous tension, but it doesn't really describe what I mean. Ah, you sort of have a terrible morbid internal dread, a fear of what's going to happen. You feel that any minute now your heart is going to stop or something like that, and that will be it, you know, or that you'll explode or something of this nature. And you get this sort of morbid internal dread or fear, absolutely irrational and unreasonable, not a logical thing at all, it's just a sort of feeling of terror. And then I begin to get breathless with this thing rather than breathless for the normal reasons, you know.

In view of the sometimes dire side-effects such treatment may carry, one is inevitably prompted to ask the question: Is it worth it? For example, are the consequences of long-term steroid treatment worse than the underlying disorder they are prescribed to treat? For those in Williams' (1990) study, the answer seemed to be that, in reality, patients had little choice. As one patient remarked: 'Well it's like a game of Russian roulette really isn't it? You have to take a chance, what else can you do? When your breathing's that bad you'll try anything just to get some relief.' Also, despite the side-effects, patients often stated that the advantages and benefits in terms of an improvement in their breathing out-weighed the disadvantages and drawbacks. Thus Mrs Prout, who, as we saw above, suffered multiple side-effects and complications, still stated:

> But despite all this, if anybody was to ask me should they go on steroids or crawl around breathless, I would say go on steroids. It's a catch twenty-two situation really.

Mrs Andrews, meanwhile, remarked:

> I mean I can moan about the steroids and I'd love to be off of them to lose some of me weight. But if it means going back to how I was then no way, I'll stay on the steroids, 'cause they keep me mobile. I mean, without them I don't think I'd be able to move.

Hospitalisation and rehabilitation

Another important aspect of therapeutic intervention, of course, concerns the hospitalisation of COAD patients. Despite the fact that hospitalisation is generally regarded as an unwelcome event in most people's lives, for those in acute respiratory distress it may none the less represent a welcome source of comfort, respite and relief. As Mr Thompson remarked:

> Well, I must admit that last time I was very glad to get there, very glad indeed, in that I was hoping for a bit of relief, and I got it. But I mean, nobody likes going into hospital. However, having got there, I mean I must admit that they're all very charming up there and they make life very, very easy. I mean you've all heard the old cliché about the medical staff and all the rest of it, and it's all quite true, they are brilliant. . . . So I mean I was very glad to get into the hospital and I felt heaps better when I came out.

Yet for some COAD patients hospitalisation is, unfortunately, a recurrent and perennial problem; particularly in the latter advanced stages of the disease. Moreover, as various studies have shown, hospitalisation is not just the product of illness severity. For example, Kaptein (1982), in a study of severe asthmatics, found that length of hospitalisation was significantly correlated with anxiety, feelings of stigma, neuroticism and hostility. Interestingly, no associations were found between length of hospitalisation and the severity or duration of the disease. Kaptein also found that those who were re-hospitalised within 6 months of their first admission were significantly more anxious, less optimistic, and felt more stigmatised than patients who were not re-hospitalised. Similarly, Jensen (1983) found that social support and life stress were better predictors of the number of hospital admissions of COAD patients than were their demographic characteristics, the severity of illness, or previous hospitalisation.

Some of those in Williams' (1990) study, for example, spoke of hospital almost as if it were their second home. As one patient remarked:

'I'm in and out of there like a yo-yo these days', whilst another appositely referred to it as like 'being stuck in a revolving door, you're no sooner out than you're back in again'. Mrs White and Mr Kerr, for example, had both been admitted three times within the last year. As Mrs White stated in the context of discussing the issue of holidays:

> Oh, we've not been on holiday for 4 years now. . . . Whenever my husband books his holiday it's fatal, I always end up in hospital. . . . We're never able to plan anything, 'cause as I say, I always seem to end up in hospital, it's infallible.

Moreover, hospitalisation can, of course, be quite a frightening event, no matter how many times a patient has previously been admitted. Thus Mrs Prout, for example, whose last hospital admission involved a stay of five and a half weeks, despite speaking very highly of the standard of care she received, still stated:

> Mind you, I'm still terrified at the thought of having to go into hospital. Well, it's stupid really, but I think everybody's the same when you're going into hospital . . . you don't know exactly what's wrong with you this time, you know, how bad it is, what's going to happen to you, how long you'll be in . . . it's always a shock to me when [Dr R] says: 'You'll have to come in'. . . . It's always such a shock to me, although I'm not well, you know, and I know I should be getting medical care of some sort.

A final important aspect of medical care, of course, concerns the rehabilitation of COAD patients. Whilst little has been done on the *experiential* aspects of rehabilitation from the perspective of COAD sufferers themselves, various studies have attempted to evaluate the effectiveness of particular rehabilitation programmes. For example, the efficacy of a four-week rehabilitation programme involving twenty-one male hospital patients was assessed by Agle *et al.* (1973) and Baum *et al.* (1973). The programme included routine medical management, breathing re-training/therapy, graduated exercise, group therapy sessions twice a week and voluntary counselling concerning both social and vocational aspects of life. Patients were followed on a monthly basis and then were re-evaluated after one year. Interestingly, in addition to the lessening of 'crippling psychologic symptoms', they also found that 'sustained improvement in function (ability to perform activities of daily living) can occur in some patients *without* demonstrable improvement in physiologic measures' (quoted in Dudley *et al.* 1980: 415–16). They also suggest that their patients' 'increased confidence in their ability to control their symptoms' might be partially responsible for the 'marked decrease in the number of hospital admissions' following the programme. Indeed, other research also suggests that physical training facilitates an improvement in respiratory muscle function and thus reduces dyspnoea, even when physiological measures of lung function have not changed.

Agle *et al.* (1973) found seven factors in their programme which they believe contributed to an improvement in both the patient's functional performance and psychological status:

1 Progressive exercise leading to a decrease in unrealistic fear of activity and dyspnoea.
2 Education in self-care leading to increased autonomy in the control of symptoms.
3 Staff attitudes stressing that the patient is worth the effort.
4 The setting of realistic goals leading to improved self-esteem.
5 Monthly follow-up to consolidate gains.
6 Mutual support from group interaction.
7 The psychosocial factors within the patient that lead to strong motivation.

(Agle *et al.* 1973, quoted in Dudley *et al.* 1980: 416)

Moreover, McSweeny and Labuhn discuss a programme devised by the American Lung Association, which includes

didactic lectures concerning the psychosocial effects of [COAD] and how to cope with them, and structured group exercises for patients with the disease and their families. This program puts a particular emphasis on 'depersonalizing' the emotional effects of [COAD] by attributing them to the disease process and teaching patients how to maximize access to activities that would yield psychological reinforcement.

(1990: 412)

Furthermore, Rosser *et al.* (1983), in another interesting study, examined the outcome of various forms of psychotherapy with sixty-five COAD patients. Whilst the group receiving treatment from a medical nurse without any formal training in psychotherapy experienced considerable relief of dyspnoea, they tended to undergo less psychodynamic change. In contrast, psychiatric symptoms, as measured by the General Health Questionnaire, were reduced in those receiving 'supportive' but not 'analytic' psychotherapy.

Finally, there have also been attempts to establish the contribution of various 'psychosocial assets' (e.g. adequate financial and material resources, extent and quality of social support, ability to cope with life style changes and alterations, a positive attitude towards life, etc.) to the rehabilitation process (Dudley *et al.* 1980). Thus Agle *et al.* (1973), for example, found that patients who suffered from 'incapacitating psychological problems' tended to respond less favourably to rehabilitation programmes than patients without such problems. As Dudley *et al.* note, results of similar studies have shown that 'patients with high psychosocial assets protect themselves more efficiently from dangerous symptoms such as attacks of dyspnoea, carried out treatment programmes more carefully and responsibly, and generally outlived their counterparts who were lacking such skills' (1980: 415).

HOPING FOR A BREAKTHROUGH: THE INVESTMENT OF HOPE IN MODERN MEDICINE

As we have seen, the lives of the chronically sick and disabled are intimately and inextricably linked with medicine. Consequently, it is perhaps understandable that patients may look to medicine for the 'solution' to their problems; investing hope in the possibility of a medical breakthrough or a panacea in the future. Indeed, the attempt to maintain such hope, a candle of optimism flickering precariously in the wind of their malaise, may represent an important aspect of their attempts to cope with their illness. Alternatively, faced with the limited ability of orthodox medicine to help, the chronically ill may turn to various alternative forms of healing in order to 'cure their ills'.

In Williams' (1990) study, for example, some patients alluded to the possibility of a heart and lung transplant; sometimes jokingly, realising their chances were slim, yet often with a serious undertone. For example:

Mr Bush: My only hope's a lung transplant. I was reading about it in the paper the other week, about a man who had one and he was 54. I spoke to the wife about it.
Mrs Bush: Yes, why can't he have one of them?
Mr Bush: Yes, you only need one good lung don't you? That's the only solution, my only hope.

For those who maintained a glimmer of hope in the possibility of having a heart and lung transplant, the realisation that this was not possible could be a devastating blow, especially if the patient's hopes had been built up by actually having been considered for one. This, unfortunately, was the case for Mrs White. Her hopes for a heart and lung transplant had been dashed, owing, she claimed, to the 'adhesions' she had in her chest. As she stated:

Well, I was very disappointed. I know it sounds silly, but I was actually looking forward to it. After all, what did I have to lose? Actually, to be quite honest with you, I was a bit annoyed that we had to wait so long for an answer as it gave me more time to build my hopes up, all to no avail. It was a terrific blow, terrible blow, I felt as though they'd pulled the rug right out from under my feet so as to speak. I mean I know they would have done it if they could, but it doesn't stop that feeling of devastation does it? I'm still hoping they might actually come up with a way of getting around this adhesions problem. I mean they're coming up with new ideas all the time aren't they? It's the only hope I've got really. I'm hoping they're not just going to forget about me. That's the only thing I think I've got to hope for now, 'cause I know I'm not going to get any better.

Others expressed hope of future medical breakthroughs such as a new 'wonder drug'. Thus Mr Thompson remarked:

I mean the other thing, of course, is that at the back of your mind you're always convinced that someone will come up with some bright idea, or some new drug or something, that will help solve the problem. I mean what with advances in medical science in recent years I think we're doing better. And so, you know, from that point of view, there's always that chance that, ah, we might do better still.

Finally, some had actually tried alternative forms of medicine or therapy in an attempt to find a solution to their problems. For example, Mr Bush had, at one point in his illness career, become very disillusioned and critical of the medical care he was receiving. Consequently, he had turned to 'faith healing' for a solution to his problems. As he stated:

Well, I was at a low ebb then, I felt very depressed . . . I mean at one point, in desperation, I even went to a spiritual healer . . . I tried faith healing on the recommendation of somebody whose parents had been and they had felt well again. So I went a couple of times, perhaps it was curiosity, I don't know, when you're desperate you'll try anything. But anyway, it didn't work for me, I guess I didn't have the faith [laughs].

Such accounts highlight not only the crucial role which medicine plays in the lives of the chronically sick, together with the hopes, sentiments and aspirations which patients invest in medicine and medical science, but also the sense of disappointment and devastation felt when such expectations and hopes are dashed. Medicine, in short, is at one and the same time a fountain of hope and a font of despair.

Chapter 4

Practical problems of daily life

As Blaxter (1976) suggests, the meaning of disability is spun out of the myriad web of problems it creates in the lives of the disabled and their families. One of the most basic and fundamental aspects of living with disability concerns the practical problems it creates in daily life. Seemingly mundane, taken-for-granted, tasks and activities of daily life suddenly become problematic; obstacles which have to be faced, negotiated and tackled on a daily basis with reduced resources. As Locker puts it:

> To the non-disabled person many, if not all activities of daily living are non-problematic; they are simply taken for granted, performed with hardly any awareness that they are being performed at all. This contrasts vividly with the experience of people disabled in some way. To them some, and frequently all, activities of everyday life are a problem and continually challenge energy, ingenuity and character. . . . At first glance, few of these problems appear to be major ones; nevertheless, they can have a significant impact on life chances. . . . Even when of little significance individually, an accumulation of such problems can be devastating. . . . Consequently, getting through the day becomes an achievement in itself and usually all that available time and energy will allow.
>
> (1983: 70)

Faced with such problems, disabled people are forced into having to devise a variety of strategies – involving themselves and others, and drawing upon practical, material, financial and social resources – in order to help them cope and get through their days: strategies which may have to be modified or adapted according to changing contexts and circumstances. Consequently, as Locker states: 'Over time the person comes to think ahead, to anticipate problems and to appreciate the fact that ordinary everyday activities need to be meticulously planned. "Thinking it out" becomes the order of the day' (1983: 71). Yet disability, of course, varies in degree and severity. Consequently the degree to which it creates practical problems of daily life may similarly vary, though the relationship is not necessarily linear, instead being influenced by a variety of other factors. Hence, it is first to a discussion of the nature and extent of disability and quality of life impairment experienced in COAD that this chapter turns, before then going on to flesh out in more substantive detail, from sufferers' and their families' own perspectives, the precise *meaning* of these facts and figures when viewed in the context of their daily lives.

DISABILITY AND QUALITY OF LIFE IMPAIRMENT IN COAD: AN OVERVIEW

As discussed in Chapters one and two, the impairment and irreversible damage which COAD causes to the lungs and respiratory system results in a paucity of oxygen intake and thus a (major) reduction in energy supply. Consequently, patients become breathless on exertion – or more colloquially 'short of breath' – and the predominant problem revolves around getting enough oxygen to furnish the energy requirements necessary for the accomplishment of everyday tasks and activities (Fagerhaugh 1975). Indeed, as Jones states, there exists a very close relationship between breathlessness and the degree of physical disability a COAD sufferer experiences:

> Breathlessness lies at the heart of disability owing to lung disease since it is that which limits exercise performance ... [it] is clearly an important source of both *inter* and *intra*-patient variability and the link between lung disease and resulting disability. Factors responsible for it are still very poorly understood, but they constitute a major unknown quantity between objective measures of disease and subjective perceptions of distress and disability.
>
> (1988: 239–40)

Yet, as Williams (1989a, b) has noted, the assessment of disability and quality of life in relation to COAD tends to have been a relatively neglected area in comparison with the research on the emotional status of COAD patients.

Barstow (1974), in her study of COAD patients, found major 'style of living' changes had occurred which included alterations in bathing, grooming, dressing, eating, sleeping and mobility. Thus the mode of dress was altered so that clothing could easily be slipped on and off; food intake was decreased due to the fact that over-distension of the stomach affects diaphragmatic breathing; whilst sleep disruptions owing to cough, dyspnoea and restlessness were common. Another study, by Hanson (1982), involved a questionnaire survey of eleven areas of social role functioning and activities of daily living such as employment, self-care, home/personal business, marriage, care of grandchildren and dependency on others. Hanson also found that COAD had a generally negative impact across all the categories covered within her study. Similarly, in Sexton and Monro's (1988) study of women with COAD, it was found that when compared to a control group of women without a chronic illness, not only did the women with COAD have lower perceived health status, higher levels of subjective stress and lower levels of life satisfaction, they also experienced greater problems in daily living such as dyspnoea and fatigue, restricted household and social activities, loneliness and depression.

McSweeny and colleagues (1982) attempted systematically to assess life quality and psychosocial functioning, utilising the Sickness Impact Profile (SIP), a quality of life instrument designed for the general population. They found COAD patients to be impaired with respect to age-matched community controls on all dimensions. Scales particularly affected appeared to include household management, physical mobility, sleep and rest, social interactions, and recreation and pastimes. In contrast, body care and movement, eating and communication were less affected. It was also found that many of the patients with COAD showed neuro-psychological impairments suggestive of cerebral dysfunction. As Grant and Heaton note: 'It should be emphasised that these substantial disabilities were observed amongst persons who were not hospitalised for their disorders but who remained ambulatory', therefore alerting physicians to the 'major disturbance in day-to-day living that COAD can produce' (1985: 367).

McSweeny *et al.* (1982) also examined the relationship between quality of life and a range of other disease-related and socio-demographic variables. In particular they found a strong relationship between their quality of life measures and COAD patients' age, socio-economic status, neuro-psychological status and exercise capability. A weaker, yet statistically significant, relationship was found to exist between quality of life and various physiological measures of COAD such as spirometry and oxygen transportation. These findings found further support in Prigatano *et al.*'s (1984) study of mildly hypoxaemic patients. They also found that neuro-psychological functioning, exercise capability and pulmonary function variables related more strongly to the physical than the psychosocial aspects of life quality as measured by the SIP. In contrast, mood and emotional status, as measured by the Minnesota Multiphasic Personality Inventory (MMPI) and the Profile of Mood States (POMS), were more strongly related to the psychosocial aspects of life quality on the SIP. As McSweeny and Labuhn remark: 'These findings demonstrate some of the complex interrelationships that exist between various aspects of quality of life, as well as between quality of life and other spheres of functioning in chronic obstructive pulmonary disease' (1990: 407–8).

Similar results were also found in Williams' study (1990, Williams and Bury 1989a, b), which utilised the British equivalent of the SIP – the Functional Limitations Profile (FLP) – in order to assess levels of physical disability and quality of life impairment in COAD. Again, as Table 4.1 shows, it was found that COAD patients tended to suffer considerable limitations over a broad range of categories of the FLP. Areas particularly affected included household management (men tending to score lower than women on this dimension: p <.001), ambulation, sleep and rest, recreation and pastimes, and work (men tending to score higher than women on this dimension: p <.03).

Table 4.1 Disability and quality of life impairment in COAD*

FLP category		Mean %
1	Work	42
2	Recreation and pastimes	40
3	Household management	35
4	Sleep and rest	32
5	Ambulation	28
6	Alertness	25
7	Mobility	23
8	Social interaction	20
9	Emotional behaviour	20
10	Body care and movement	15
11	Communication	9
12	Eating	5
	Global physical disability	20
	Global psychosocial	19
	Overall FLP	22

* Scores range (theoretically) from 0 to 100 per cent. In the Lambeth disability study, community controls (i.e. men and women in the following two age bands: 25–64, 65–77 yrs) scored ≤5 per cent on all FLP categories (Patrick and Peach 1989).

As these findings serve to highlight, the predominant type of disability stemming from COAD tends to be locomotor-based with little or no loss of manual dexterity. Thus it differs from musculo-skeletal conditions such as rheumatoid arthritis, where one may perhaps expect higher FLP scores in areas such as 'body care and movement'.

In addition, Williams' study (1990, Williams and Bury 1989a, b) also found that spirometric measures of lung function were only weakly related to dyspnoea, physical disability and psychosocial aspects of quality of life. Guyatt *et al.* (1987) report similar findings in their study, in which the severity of COAD patients' airflow obstruction was not significantly related to their identified problems or quality of life. Indeed, as other research shows, psychological factors such as mood, attitudes and beliefs are important predictors of exercise tolerance (Morgan *et al.* 1983a, b); suggesting that psychological variables are at least as important, if not more so, than initial ventilatory status.

Yet, important though the above findings undoubtedly are, they mean very little when considered on their own. Hence, it is to a more substantive discussion of the *meaning* of these facts and figures from sufferers' and their families' *own* perspectives, viewed within the context of their daily lives, that this chapter now turns.

PROBLEMATIC ASPECTS OF DAILY LIFE: 'INSIDERS'' ACCOUNTS

'Getting around' with COAD

As we have seen, one of the key problems for the COAD sufferer concerns the inability to get enough oxygen to furnish the energy requirements necessary for ambulation and the accomplishment of everyday tasks and activities. Hence, as Fagerhaugh (1975) suggests, it is in this respect that 'getting around' becomes a major issue and a perennial problem in COAD sufferers' lives. Fagerhaugh conceptualises the problems emphysema sufferers face in terms of the selective allocation of what she terms Basic Mobility Resources (BMRs): namely, time, energy and money, all of which are drawn upon for physical mobility and sociability. Thus in Williams' (1990) study, for example, respondents' accounts highlighted the considerably complex, indeed tortuous, planning and strategic decision-making processes involved in the allocation of their scarce resources. Mr Brown, for instance, graphically illustrated the strategic dilemmas faced and the 'gauging techniques' required when considering a sojourn to the shops:

I mean for someone like you, you don't let it cross your mind, you think 'Oh I've got to pop across the road and buy something' and off you go. But me, I've got to stop and think about the pitfalls of that same shopping expedition which, for example, might only be two, three hundred yards down the road. But I've got to stop and think: 'Is it too far for me?'; 'Can I manage it?'; 'Is it beyond me?'; 'Will I get out of my depth?'; 'Where can I rest in between?'; 'Where is it suitable where there's not too many people?', you know, 'cause you hate to draw attention to yourself, and so on. So you've got to make all these decisions before you go. You've got to stop and study, plan and judge, every movement you make. Things that once upon a time you took for granted, did unwittingly, they're problematic for me nowadays.

Mr Ash, meanwhile, stated:

Well, if you wanna do anything, you've got to continually think round what you wanna do. Whereas one time, if I wanted to do anything I'd just get up and do it, now you've gotta think: 'Well can I do it?'

Perhaps the first problems COAD sufferers face in 'getting around', however, begin at home; particularly negotiating stairs. As Barstow (1974) found in her study: 'Climbing stairs and running were given up early.' Similarly, many of those in Williams' (1990) study spoke of the difficulty and distress they encountered when negotiating stairs. As Mr King stated:

Well, in the home the biggest problem is the stairs. It's going up the stairs that's the problem, there's no trouble at all coming down the stairs. I don't know why they make stairs that go up, they should all be ones that go down [laughs]! But going up stairs, well, I just can't navigate stairs at all. You see it depends on the kind of stairs they are, you find some staircases are very steep and if they're very steep, well I can only manage three or four and then I've got to stop. But here at home there are fifteen and they are not too steep, so I can manage about ten of them and then I have to stop, once I've gone that far I'm completely beaten. I've got to stop, get rejuvenated – by that I mean wait until I get my breath and energy back – and then start again!

Faced with such problems, strategies to minimise the use of stairs may, in addition to relying on 'normal lungers', include bringing everything needed during the day down in the morning, or leaving things at the foot of the staircase and, if not too heavy, taking them all up in one go at the end of the day. As Mr King stated:

Oh well, I try to think of everything upstairs that I'm possibly going to need during the day and bring it down with me in the morning. You see, once I'm downstairs I like to stay there, 'cause it's a devil's own job getting back up again! The worst thing is when you're short of time. For instance, if I were going off to catch a bus or something like that and I had forgotten something I needed from upstairs, well if there's no one else in the house then you've had it; you've missed your bus! God I don't know how many buses and trains I must have missed over the years because of this! So you have to leave yourself plenty of time when you're going out anywhere, especially when you're in the house alone, in case you forget something. Otherwise, well the bus has gone!

Mrs Andrews, meanwhile, remarked:

I mean, you don't keep going up and down the stairs do you, you sort of work your day out don't you? For instance, I put things on the stairs so that when you do go up, you take everything with you, you know, when you've gotta go to the toilet you just take everything with you. And while you're up there you do the beds and bins and what have you, you know what I mean, I work it that way.

Other strategies of a more long-term nature may include the installation of chair-lifts, moving bedrooms downstairs, or alternatively moving to bungalows or ground-floor flats.

Of course, beyond these immediate problems of getting about inside the home, COAD sufferers also, particularly in the advanced stages of the disease, tend to experience considerable limitations in their general ambulatory capacities outside the home. In Williams' (1990) study, for example, the degree of exercise tolerance, as measured on the Fletcher Breathlessness Grading Scale (Fletcher et al. 1959), ranged from 2 (breathless when hurrying on the level/walking up a slight hill) to 5 (breathless on (un)dressing/after a few yards). For example, when asked how far she could walk, Mrs Andrews replied:

Not very far. If I go from here [her flat], downstairs . . . and I get to the corner and I walk round, there's a crossing there where I cross to go over to the shops, and I usually stand there and let the lights change a couple of times before I attempt to cross, because by then I'm out of breath. But I do make myself try and reach that point before I'll stop. I could stop earlier, sometimes I have to, you know, I don't get to the corner, I just get to the LEB and I stop and lean on the railings there. But, umh, I do try and make meself go round the corner to the crossing.

And I've got a couple of nice stopping places along there, you know, and I've got me favourite seats [laughs], they all know me along there now. There's a couple of building societies along there and they've got seats inside haven't they. So if it's a particularly rough day, then I'll go in there and I'll just wave to them behind the counter, sit on one of their chairs for ten minutes and have a puff.

Similarly Mr Bush – who rarely went out, especially on his own, claiming that 'I know I'm limited and I don't want to get out of me depth' – recounted the following story:

Well, take yesterday for example, yesterday was a nice day and so I decided to go and get the newspaper from the paper shop on the corner. . . . Well, I got half way over there and I began to feel the strain, I was caught half way, and then you begin to panic, especially if you're on your own. So I stopped and started to look up and down the street and at me watch as if I was waiting for someone. Anyway, eventually I made it to the paper shop, bought a paper and then did a bit of 'window shopping' in order to regain me strength and breath for the journey home – although to be honest with you I don't know what the hell I was looking at! And eventually I made it back home, at me own pace like, you know.

Meanwhile, Mr Doyal, who fared relatively better than some in terms of breathlessness and ambulatory capacity, stated:

On ground level I'm OK, I can just do a steady gait, you know, take it easy, at me own pace like. I've always been a fast walker, but I've learnt to control me walking and me pace now, and I manage it, you know.

Also, carrying any additional weight may, of course, make a substantial difference to the COAD sufferer's ambulatory capabilities. As Mr King remarked:

Well, for example, I might manage to go to the corner store to get something light in the way of shopping sometimes, such as a bottle of milk or a loaf of bread, but I can't manage anything heavy . . . anything I get has to be very, very light, because I can't carry anything heavy at all, any kind of additional weight surplus to requirements leaves me breathless.

Moreover, the fluidity and simultaneity of tasks, actions and activities tends to be profoundly disrupted by COAD. Whereas, for a 'normal' individual, walking whilst talking is accomplished unthinkingly and with ease, for COAD sufferers it may be a case of doing one or the other, not both. Thus Miss Bell, for example, found that when she went shopping with her friend, it was very difficult 'both to walk and talk at the same time'; Mrs White found that when caught by a sudden attack of breathlessness, she did not have the breath to speak to other people who 'flapped' around her; whilst Mr O'Riley, when out, would just wave and carry on walking if a friend or acquaintance greeted him, rather than attempt to hold a conversation.

It is in such contexts that, as Fagerhaugh suggests, a basic mobility-related strategy of 'routing' takes place:

> The process by which all persons, whether ill or healthy, deal with problems of mobility is by routing. The dimensions involved are: 1) anticipation of the number and types of activities in terms of available BMRs; 2) judgements whether to delete or postpone some activities, or to condense activities by combining several activities; 3) sequential ordering of activities in terms of the importance, distance, time and energy involved in each activity, as well as anticipation of possible obstacles.
>
> (1975: 103)

For COAD sufferers, routing is essential in order to avoid the consequences of over-exertion and anxiety (Fagerhaugh 1975). Hence, if they are to maximise their mobility potentials, COAD sufferers must learn to think and plan ahead regarding the most convenient routes and modes of travel. Consequently, they must take into account factors such as the time and energy requirements involved, together with the costs and benefits of the various modes of travel available; the local terrain and geography; whether or not there are convenient stopping places or 'puffing stations' *en route* when travelling by foot; and, finally, the weather and climatic conditions.

Many of those in Williams' (1990) study spoke of how they had found various convenient and, perhaps more importantly, inconspicuous stopping places or 'puffing stations' when on their peripatetic jaunts. Thus, garden walls, park benches, chairs in shops, railings, lamp-posts, bus stops and telephone boxes, together with a frequently alluded to policy of 'window shopping' or 'looking as if I'm waiting for someone', were amongst the range of locations and strategies mentioned for 'recouping', 'rejuvenating' and 'regaining' oneself when in public. For example, Mrs Andrews, as mentioned above, had a 'couple of nice stopping places' and her 'favourite seats' *en route*, Miss Bell had her own 'set little secluded places where I can stop for a rest', and Mr Doyal stated:

Yeah well, I've got gardens and seats there which I can stop and rest on . . . they're deposited all round the place. So I walk a short distance and then I can sit on a seat or a wall till I get to the main road . . . and that short stretch, I can walk down to the shops from there. But when I come back, especially if I've got stuff to carry, I have to rest on the first seat, and then I'll walk to the next one and have another rest . . . 'Cause the going's not so bad, it's downhill, but coming back, I've got to negotiate that hill. Coming back, somedays I've gotta rest twice before I can get to me first seat. I stand up against the wall, or I'll sit on a low level wall outside somebody's house.

Hills may also come to represent (sometimes insuperable) problems. As Mr King remarked:

I can't go up hills, they leave me dead on my feet. Well of course, if I have to go up them I'll go up them, but I'll avoid them if I can. But if it's a steep hill, I can't make it at all, if it's some sort of gradual incline then, yeah, but it's going to take me an awful long time to get there. Because sometimes, I can only take as much as three or four steps and I'll have to stop again, and it puts an awful lot of pressure on the old chest.

Miss Bell, meanwhile, whose local tube station was located at the top of a hill with a fairly steep incline, spoke of how on 'bad days' if she needed to use the tube she would catch a bus which 'goes all the way round the one-way system and stops at the top of the hill near the station'. Moreover, as discussed in Chapter two, COAD sufferers also have to contend with the effect which the weather and general climatic conditions may have on their symptoms, and hence their ambulatory and mobility-related capabilities. As Fagerhaugh states:

Emphysema patients must also weigh the weather more carefully than do normals because they must avoid catching colds. Windy weather is said to increase breathing problems. Also there is the question of avoiding a tailwind or headwind. And, of course, smog greatly increases their breathing problems.

(1975: 104)

Faced with such difficulties, it is perhaps understandable why some COAD sufferers, particularly in the advanced stages of the disease, retreat into the home and rarely venture out. Those fortunate enough to own or have access to a car may, of course, remain relatively mobile despite such problems. Yet for those who lack such a resource, the stark choice is often one of attempting to remain as mobile as possible by struggling with public transport, or of withdrawing more and more into the confines of the home.

Energy, sleep and rest

As we have seen, not only does COAD result in breathlessness on exertion, it also, through a paucity of oxygen, tends to produce a chronic shortage of energy and generalised feelings of lethargy. Thus a large proportion of COAD sufferers' time is consumed in having to rest. The vast majority of those in Williams' (1990) study, for instance, found a lack of energy a considerable problem: whilst 3 per cent rated it as only being a 'slight problem', 36 per cent rated it as a 'middling problem' and 61 per cent rated it as a 'big problem' in their daily lives. As Mr King put it:

> I have a terrible lack of energy. I get terribly, terribly tired and worn out very easily, you're always short of energy. Really it's difficult to separate the breathlessness from the lack of energy, the two are related I suppose aren't they. I mean I guess that if you can't breathe very well your body's not getting enough oxygen into the system to produce the energy you need, the two go hand in glove you see. Anyway, the upshot of it is, the bottom line, that whether it's getting up in the morning, washing or dressing, anything, you get so damned tired and breathless. . . . You get tired so easily, everything you try to do, no matter how small a task it is, it seems to drain the energy right out of you, you seem to get so tired during the day. You see I've got the energy in my head, but translating it, well that's the problem. I can imagine all the things in the world that I used to do, but when it comes to actually trying to do anything, well it just isn't there it's as simple as that.

Thus tasks and activities have to be carefully and painstakingly assessed, weighed and planned in terms of their energy requirements; how much sufferers actually feel capable of doing on the day; the number and amount of rest periods required in between; and, finally, the amount of time required to complete these tasks or activities as against other competing needs and priorities. As Mrs White put it: 'I have to think "Well, what do I feel like today, how energetic do I feel?" ' Many also spoke of the sheer volume of time which was consumed just having to rest, and of how they often found themselves dozing or nodding off during the day. As Mr Thompson stated:

Generally speaking I do sleep and have to rest quite a lot. I mean, if I do sit down during the daytime I'll inevitably fall asleep. I'll probably fall asleep in the evening as well.

Yet one of the cruel ironies of COAD concerns the fact that whilst rest is essential, the disease may also interfere considerably with the sufferer's actual ability to sleep and rest; interrupting regular sleep patterns and hence causing still further fatigue. Thus a vicious circle oftens tends to result. As Barstow found in her study:

> Changes reported . . . included going to bed earlier, alterations in the sleeping position for sleeping and less restful sleep. . . . Sleep was interrupted by cough, dyspnea or restlessness. Coping techniques included the use of drugs to alleviate the cough and dyspnea, and eating, reading or watching television for relaxation and the facilitation of sleep.
>
> (1974: 141–2)

As Table 4.1 indicates, considerable problems surrounding sleep and rest were also experienced by those in Williams' (1990) study. The main reasons cited included some or all of the following: breathlessness and coughing; the inability to sleep lying down; and, finally, as the illness progressed, a more vaguely defined inability to sleep soundly at night, perhaps due to psychological factors. Thus Mr Brown stated:

> Oh, I have trouble with my sleep. Well, for a start I have difficulty getting to sleep and so I need artificial help – either a glass of whisky before going to bed at night or I take sleeping tablets. And so, as a consequence, I never feel really refreshed after sleeping. . . . But I mean, I frequently get woken up in the night with me breathing and I often have to go on the nebuliser in the night. . . . I mean, I can be woken up anything up to three times a night breathless, sometimes it's just once and other times I can get away with it. . . . I mean I get very tired during the day and I never feel refreshed because of the difficulties I have sleeping, but I can't sleep in an armchair. And my wife, she gets tired too, 'cause she gets woken up with it all . . . you know.

Mrs McLeod, meanwhile, remarked:

> Well, getting to sleep isn't such a problem, the biggest problem is *staying* asleep. I'll just get off to sleep and I'll wake up an hour or so later very, very breathless, you know, gasping. And I'll sit there until I get me breath back and then I'll go off again. Then I'll wake up again

after about, say, two or three hours. So in a 'normal' night I'll wake up about, say, oh I don't know, three times. I mean a 'good' night for me is only being woken up once, at times it can be quite frightening.

As Mr Brown's account highlights, not only do sleeping problems affect the sufferer, they may also cause considerable problems for their families, particularly the spouse. Faced with such problems and difficulties, some had taken to sleeping in separate bedrooms so as not to disturb their spouses 'too much' during a 'bad night'. Thus Mrs Charlton, for instance, who still worked full-time, had taken to sleeping in the spare bedroom:

Mr Charlton: Oh yeah, I don't sleep, no, I'm awake the whole night really to be honest with you. Well, to be honest, I doze off during the day time, I doze off for about ten minutes, quarter of an hour. But at night time, I just can't sleep at night. . . . And the wife, she sleeps in the spare bedroom nowadays. See she has a hard job sleeping 'cause I cough a lot during the night. As soon as I start a coughing fit, she'll holler out if I'm all right see.

Mrs Charlton: Yeah, I'll get up for him then and see if he's all right and I'll walk about with him.

Mr Charlton: Well, she's got to work, I mean it's not fair to her really. But when I'm bad she wakes up and she'll say: 'Are you all right, do you want any help?' And if I want her I'll say: 'Yes', or she might get up and make me a cuppa tea or something like that, you know.

Mrs Charlton: Yeah, 'cause I know when it's gonna happen now, I can sort of sense it now, 'cause I mean it happens so much. . . . But it can't be helped can it, I mean he can't help it can he? We both really need a few good nights' sleep.

It is factors such as these which further add to the physical and psychosocial problems and difficulties of living and coping with COAD. As one sufferer aptly remarked: 'There's no peace, no let up with this thing, you can't even escape when you go to bed at night, it's with you twenty-four hours a day!'

Personal care

Another important area of people's day-to-day existence, of course, concerns what are perhaps the most basic, fundamental tasks of daily life, ones which traditionally have constituted key criteria in defining 'dependence' and 'independence' in activities of daily living (ADL): namely, those pertaining to personal care. As Barstow (1974) found in her study, in the early stages, an increase in the length of time required to perform such activities was reported. However, as the pulmonary disability increased other problems emerged:

> The morning toilet and dressing were often done in stages with rest pauses interspersed; some patients required the assistance of others. Head level activities, such as brushing teeth, shaving, and combing hair, were particularly tiring. Showers 'suffocated' the person and baths were 'tiresome'. . . . The mode of dress was altered in favour of less restrictive clothing that was easily slipped on and off. . . . Stooping and leaning over also compromised breathing, so laced shoes were given up in favour of slip-ons. . . . Lying down after a heavy meal restricted breathing, since an overdistended stomach presses against the diaphragm and makes inspiration more difficult, so food intake was decreased, particularly at the evening meal. . . . Lifting, pushing, pulling, and stooping required high energy expenditure and tasks involving these movements were done slowly, if at all.
>
> (1974: 141–2)

Similarly, although the majority of those in Williams' (1990) study could accomplish most tasks independently, they were far from unproblematic. Even simple tasks like washing, shaving and (un)dressing left some patients breathless and worn out. As Mr King averred:

> just getting out of bed first thing in the morning and washing my face and hands, the bare rudiments, takes me about twenty minutes. That's fast, and that's only washing my face and hands, as I say the bare rudiments, that's all.

Similarly, Mr Charlton stated:

> Well, I can wash meself, as I said, if I take me time, but I do get short of breath on washing, oh yeah, terrible. Washing meself and moving me arms and head and all that, you know, or shaving, me arms seem to ache, you know what I mean.

Concerning (un)dressing, Mr Ash remarked:

> Umh, it's a slow job dressing. . . . It's a slow job usually, so's getting undressed. I'll start getting dressed or undressed and then I'll have to stop for a little while to get me breath back, you know, if I get too bad

I'll go on the oxygen, but, ah, usually I tend to keep off it as much as I can. . . . You see I'll do a little bit and then I'll stop for a rest, do something else, then I'll come back to getting dressed again. I don't do it all in one go usually, I never really try it all in one go these days 'cause I would lose me breath straight away. So I tend to do it in stages 'cause I find it's easiest for me.

And Mrs McLeod stated:

It varies, some days it's harder than others. Sometimes I manage to get dressed pretty easily. But other days I'll put me bra and knicks on and have to sit on the bed until I get me breath back, I'll have a bit of a rest before I go on and do a bit more, you know, it varies from day-to-day. And I mean I have to sit on the bed or settee and lift me feet up to put me tights and shoes on, or I'll sit on the floor and do it, you know. But I mean I wear slippers indoors and I don't bother with tights so, you know. And I mean I buy a lot of slip-on shoes for going out, which helps, you know.

Bathing and showering may also present problems and difficulties for those with COAD. For those with severe disability, just getting in and out of the bath and attempting to wash oneself tends to leave them breathless, hence help is often required. For others the steam of the bath or shower can be a problem, leaving them short of breath. Consequently steam production has to be carefully controlled and minimised by not having the water too hot and leaving doors and windows open. Of course, once out of the bath, the act of drying oneself off can also leave the COAD sufferer both considerably breathless and drained of energy. Thus either such tasks have to be taken very slowly, or else the help of others is sought. As Mr King remarked:

Well it's quite a job, even taking a shower, 'cause any activity I do, even just washing myself, it takes energy, you're expending energy and so it leaves you short of breath, even towelling yourself off afterwards. And you have to watch out for the steam, you can't have it too hot 'cause the steam'll leave you breathless. So it's quite a task nowadays having a shower.

Mr Kerr, meanwhile, who did not possess a shower, required help in bathing:

Mrs Kerr: I have to help him get in and out of the bath and I help wash him once he's in there, you know.

Mr Kerr: Yeah, 'cause you still get breathless once you're in there see, what with the washing and the steam and what have you. But I try not to have it too hot and I don't go in there until she's got rid of some of the steam, you know, she'll leave the door and the windows open for a while – well I leave the door open all the time to get rid of the steam and let some air in. . . . And when I get out the wife has to help dry me off, the wife does that for me, I couldn't manage it, I'd get too breathless see.

In view of these problems, some had resorted to wrapping themselves in large, absorbent, towelling dressing gowns in order to avoid the necessity of having to dry themselves off. Another strategy mentioned by some was to have a bath or shower last thing at night, as having it first thing in the morning left them drained of energy for the rest of the day. Moreover, this also, of course, obviated the necessity of having to get dressed again!

Household management

Woven inextricably into the texture of everyday life are the tasks, duties and responsibilities of household management. As Table 4.1 shows, COAD sufferers tend to experience considerable disability in this realm of daily life, although, perhaps unsurprisingly, women tend to score higher than men within this domain (p <.001). Many of those in Williams' (1990) study, for example, discussed the problems and difficulties they faced regarding household management. Some had virtually been forced to give them up altogether, whilst others still managed to struggle on, engaged in fighting the symbolic battle between 'dependence' and 'independence' with remarks such as 'I wouldn't give in', or 'I refuse to be beaten, however long it takes me and however hard it is.' For instance Mrs Andrews, who was widowed, gave the following account of the problems and difficulties she faced regarding housework:

Well, I still do all me own cooking, washing and ironing, yes. I do the cooking. Umh, I gotta washing machine so that's OK. . . . Umh, I do me ironing, it's a bit of an effort nowadays but I still manage to do it, 'cause there's less for me to do now anyway. I don't know how I'd cope now if the four of us were still here [laughs]. But I still do manage to do it, slowly of course. I usually have a little stop and a sit down and then I get up again and have another go. Making beds is, oh that's terrible, I can't, I'm no good with beds . . . and vacuuming, that's absolutely awful [laughs], I don't know why, I suppose it's the effort of pushing the thing around, but I cannot vacuum, it's really terrible . . . I seem to be using all me energy in doing it. And so, of course, I gotta keep turning it off and having a rest. And by the time I've gone round here it's took me about two and a half hours just to do this living room. And I sit here and I think 'Thank God that's done', you know, and you'd think I'd just scrubbed the house from top to bottom [laughs]. Oh it's awful, it really is murder.

Mrs White, meanwhile, remarked:

I do get very frustrated . . . the fact that I can't do *what* I want, *how* I want, *when* I want, it's a very frustrating illness. I mean my home, well I know my husband tries but it's not like it used to be, not how *I* would like it to be. Silly little things that used to be real chores suddenly become important and niggle you. I mean the oven needs cleaning, the cupboards need cleaning out and the freezer needs defrosting. These are things I can't do anymore and I don't like to ask my husband. I know he'd do it, but it's not fair on him is it, he's already got enough to do, he hasn't got the time. The most frustrating thing is when you go to start something but you can't finish it, which often happens. I get set into doing something and have to give up, that's very frustrating indeed, you feel beaten and I don't like being beaten.

As both Barstow (1974) and Fagerhaugh (1975) found in their studies, faced with such problems, two major coping techniques concern the 'simplification' and 'pacing' of activities:

Both of these concepts could be subsumed under 'planning ahead to maximize economy of effort'. Many activities involving physical effort can be simplified or 'resting pauses' can be planned so that the activities can continue to be performed by the patient with emphysema.

(Barstow 1974: 141)

Moreover, it is in contexts such as these that 'standards' have to be 'lowered'; what Weiner (1975) terms a process of downward 'spiral re-normalisation'. As Mrs White put it:

Take the housework for instance, you just have to lower your standards, lower your expectations, you know, accept things that once you wouldn't have dreamed of accepting; learn to live with the fact that you can't keep your house as you'd like to; and learn to accept and be grateful for what other people are doing for you, even if it's not being done quite how you'd like!

Shopping may also prove problematic for some or all of the following reasons: limited mobility; the inability to carry heavy shopping bags; the encumbrance and embarrassment of medical aids and appliances such as oxygen cylinders when in public; fear of being in crowded, busy places which may trigger an attack of dyspnoea; and, finally, the fear or risk of picking up a chest infection. Many of those in Williams' (1990) study who were married spoke of how their spouses did all the shopping nowadays; a situation which for many male sufferers did not represent a significant change, compared to the position when it was the wife who was ill. In contrast, those who lived alone either had to rely on friends, relatives or social services for help, or were forced to struggle on their own as best they could, a situation which was particularly problematic if they lacked access to a car. Mrs McLeod's husband, for example, had now taken over responsibility for the shopping, which, being busy at work all week, he had to do at the weekends. In contrast Miss Bell, who lived alone, had a friend who came round once a week with a trotter. They would then go to the shops together to get her main weekly goods, which her friend had to carry up the stairs to her flat as there was no lift in the building. Meanwhile Mr and Mrs Pinter, who were both disabled and did not own a car, had to struggle to the local shops and manage as best they could between them. As Mr Pinter put it:

> Like the shopping, there's bags to carry, and so I carry them. We've gotta trolley, but what's a trolley, five minutes and it's full up, you know what I mean. So you know, I mean you've everything else on top. But we both can't walk for miles, so we have to struggle all in one go to bring it back home again.

Similarly, as COAD progresses, household maintenance and repairs may prove increasingly difficult if not impossible. Indeed, many of the men in Williams' (1990) study who claimed to have been 'DIY enthusiasts' in the past said that they had now been forced, in the face of their illness, to give up. Mr Thomas, for example, described the problems and difficulties he faced with the aid of a botanical metaphor:

> And I mean decorating, that's another big problem. The kitchen and hall want doing, sooner or later it's all got to be done including the outside front and back. Once upon a time I would have done it meself, but I can't do it now. I'll either have to pay for it to be done . . . or else rely on the goodwill and charity of others, Christ knows who though! I mean, things I used to be able to do for meself, and things that when I was working I could have afforded to have done, will just have to go

to pot now. How can I put it [pauses]. To me this house is like a plant that's beginning to wilt and die slowly but surely around me, and as a man who used to do a bit in the house I find that very depressing, you know what I mean.

In contrast Mr Ash had, to a certain extent, anticipated such problems and strategically planned ahead:

You see, everything that's been done in this house has been done for a purpose. There's washable wallpaper that just needs sponging down now and the pine cladding on them walls over there and on the ceiling, that'll be all right for years. And I mean, the rest's just emulsion see. Even them doors have got clear wood varnish on 'em and the staircase is emulsioned. It's all been done for a purpose, you know, 'cause I anticipated this would happen. So when I last did it five years ago, I was planning ahead like, you know what I mean.

Despite being a recommended form of recreation for COAD sufferers (Petty and Nett 1984), gardening may also prove problematic as the illness progresses. As Mr Thompson remarked:

Well I might sometimes mow the lawn but my wife usually comes out and takes over. . . . I mean there's a lot I'd like to do but the fact is I can't any more, gardening defeats me. I mean I've done all the mechanisation of the garden that I possibly can do. I've even got a little cultivator to dig the little bit of garden that we do use, I mean it's ridiculous really. But despite all that, gardening still really defeats me.

Moreover, for the disabled individual, the fact of having to sit back and watch others do things in the house or garden which once they were able to do, and took pride in doing, themselves may be a profoundly frustrating and depressing experience; one which has ramifications at both a practical and symbolic level, serving as a continual reminder of their physical limitations and further undermining their self-image. As Mr Ash put it:

for instance, the fellow next door put the fence up last week. He said to me: 'Well you can't do it so I'll do it.' So I had to sit there and watch him do it. And I ended up getting more frustrated watching him do it than I probably would have done trying to do it myself, 'cause I couldn't go out there and help, you know. I ended up getting more agitated and more out of breath just watching him, than I probably would have been if I'd actually gone out there myself and tried to lend a hand. And when I see her [his wife] out there doing the garden or a bit of decorating, it upsets me, I get a bit short tempered and breathless then, I don't like it.

Housing

Another important issue for the chronically sick and disabled, of course, concerns housing. Sixteen per cent of those in Williams' (1990) study stated that they had housing problems related to their illness or disability. These included: a lack of adequate heating; cold, damp housing likely to exacerbate respiratory symptoms; needing a ground-floor flat or accommodation without any stairs to climb; or, finally, a need to move from polluted (inner) city environments on grounds of respiratory ill-health. For example, Mrs Andrews' main housing problem revolved around the fact that she lived in a council flat situated on the top floor, with seven flights of stairs to climb and no lift service. She had applied for re-housing almost a year and a half ago – with a doctor's letter in support of her application – but had heard nothing. She claimed that even going *down* the stairs was a problem and that this restricted still further her ability to get out and about, especially when she was having a 'bad' day. As she stated:

> there are days I just don't make no attempt to go out no more, even if I've got an appointment somewhere, I'll just phone up and say: 'I'm very very sorry, but I'm just not well.' Because I can go out and I can go down the stairs, that's OK, that's not too bad, but the problem comes when I come back, it's just so unbearable. I mean, you've gotta come back up half a dozen or so of the stairs at a time and then you've gotta sit on the stairs, and I mean they're not very nice are they!

Mr Pinter described his flat, which was not centrally heated or double-glazed, as 'a devil to keep warm in the winter'. Consequently, he had to make do with an electric fire in the living room, oil-fired radiators elsewhere, and an ingenious form of double-glazing based on cling film in order to stop the draughts! Mr O'Riley, meanwhile, complained of dampness:

> Well it applies to two or three of the rooms actually, they get very damp in the winter time . . . and I mean it can't be doing me chest any good can it, makes you wonder, you know . . . it doesn't do me any good at all I don't suppose.

In contrast, Mr Stannard had applied on grounds of respiratory ill-health to move out of London to the coast, where, as he put it, 'the air is better'.

THE MANAGEMENT OF TIME

Throughout this chapter, reference has continually been made to the crucial issue of time and its management in the lives of the chronically ill and disabled. As we have seen, at one level, time is a vital, yet all too scarce, resource in the lives of the chronically sick and disabled. Thus even simple, everyday, mundane things take an inordinately greater period of time to accomplish. Indeed, as Strauss states:

> Even just handling one's symptoms or the consequences of having symptoms may take so much time that life is taken up with handling them. This can be seen very strikingly; . . . the amount of time spent resting by emphysema sufferers whilst in the midst of activities or tasks – with time fragmented or stretched out – is enormous.
>
> (1975: 45)

And Mr King graphically remarked:

> Time is essential, it's a must, you have to allocate much more time to any-thing and everything you do. So time, time you've got to allow for, you've got to allow yourself plenty of time because . . . if I don't I'm dead. I get so short of breath trying to hurry I can't do anything in the end. Even if I put my jacket on in a hurry, that will make me breathless, so I'm better off taking my time. Trying to do things at a 'normal' pace is beyond me now, it's counter-productive, 'cause I end up completely para-lysed, good for nothing. So as I say, time's an essential commodity for me nowadays. The only trouble is that, because of the illness, there appears to be much less of it because things take me so damned long to do!

Yet paradoxically, at one and the same time, the enforced limitations imposed by COAD may mean that there is too much time and that, consequently, it appears to pass very slowly or drag. As Strauss states: 'Among the consequences of too much time are boredom, decreased social skills, family strains, negative impact on identity and even physical deterioration' (1975: 44). As Miss Bell, who lived alone, remarked:

> Oh time does drag sometimes, it can be a very long day, especially when you're not feeling too good, you're inclined to feel a bit more sorry for yourself then. Or in winter months when it's cold and wet outside and you're stuck at home indoors, you think to yourself: 'Oh dear, what a long day it is, nobody cares', you know. But then I try and think, I say to meself: 'There's plenty of people worse off than me', you know, haven't got anybody. So I try and cheer meself up that way.

It is in this sense that, as Strauss (1975) suggests, chronic illness may result in a profound multi-dimensional sense of temporal disruption: one in which time has to be completely and continually re-ordered. Hence, a form of 'temporal juggling' occurs:

> The basic temporal problems – too much time, too little time, scheduling and timing – involve patients and their agents (assisting, controlling, protecting, caretaking and so forth) in a delicately balanced game of temporal juggling.
>
> (1975: 46)

Such temporal disruption adds a further subtle layer of disadvantage to the experience and challenge which living with and adjusting to a chronic disabling illness on a daily basis poses.

THE PROCESS OF 'BECOMING DISABLED'

This chapter has attempted to elucidate and touch upon a number of important themes and issues pertaining to the lives of COAD sufferers: the problematic character of what hitherto was accomplished unthinkingly with ease; the inordinate amount of time consumed in accomplishing mundane tasks of daily life; the struggle to retain a semblance of 'independence', together with the feelings surrounding the threat or reality of 'dependence'. Yet all of these processes lead, via their varied and tortuous routes, in one and the same direction: namely, the process of what Locker has referred to as 'becoming disabled':

> Learning how to pace and cope with greatly diminished resources is part of a broader process which may be referred to as becoming disabled. People with chronic illness not only have to learn how to manage symptoms, medical crises, and therapeutic regimens (Strauss 1975), they also have to learn to live with physical limitations. This involves discovering new ways of performing everyday tasks and discovering which tasks cannot be done or should not be attempted.
>
> (1983: 40–1)

As Locker goes on to note, the process of becoming disabled is perhaps facilitated in two main ways:

> firstly, by the advice given by doctors [other health care professionals] or co-sufferers and secondly, by personal experience. It is largely by trial and error that the boundaries of activity are defined and periodically reaffirmed and meaning given to advice previously provided.
>
> (1983: 41)

Yet as Blaxter (1976) has suggested, disability is a *social* rather than clinical fact; the relationship between the two being far from clear-cut. This is further compound by the fact that, as Chapter six discusses, COAD is a largely 'invisible' disease in which the resulting disability is less immediately evident than in certain other chronic conditions. For example, there were some in Williams' (1990) study whose illness and disability were considerable, but who rejected the suggestion that the label applied to them in any way. In contrast, others who were relatively better off by comparison appeared to be somewhat 'overwhelmed' by their illness and disability and hence were more ready to accept that the label did indeed apply to them now. This serves to reinforce the point made above that becoming disabled is a *social* process which should not be lost sight of by those concerned with the clinical care and rehabilitation of COAD sufferers.

Chapter 5

Problems of work and income

For many chronically sick and disabled people, the struggle to maintain an economically active and independent role in the labour force is considerable. Similarly, the loss of or final decision to give up work in the wake of a chronic disabling illness is equally problematic; one which may have implications at the practical, material, financial, social and symbolic levels. As Locker notes:

> As far as disabled persons are concerned, their occupational careers are likely to be structured by a number of factors, including the nature of the illness and the strategies required to manage it, the velocity of the illness trajectory, the nature of the work and the possibility that it can be reorganised in the face of disability, and the tolerance of workmates and employers.
>
> (1983: 98)

These factors, together with the predominantly manual working-class background of COAD sufferers – who may have few skills to offer in the labour market and possess a limited ability to re-train – combine to produce considerable occupational, financial and social disadvantage for both sufferers and their families. Hence it is to a more detailed and substantive discussion of some of the many problems which COAD sufferers face in relation to work and income that this chapter now turns.

PROBLEMATIC ASPECTS OF WORK

> One of the first roles to change, in response to less energy is the *role of the working man*. Emphysema is an episodic, expensive illness that attacks its victims in their fourth and fifth decades of life when the working man would ordinarily be at the peak of his career, and when his responsibilities to his family are at a high level. . . . If the patient's

job is not too physically tiring, he may continue his work; otherwise he may have to retire. If he is a bricklayer and no longer has the energy to lift bricks, his role as a working man will change.

(Barstow 1974: 139; my emphasis)

The predominant features of COAD and its sequelae which, either singularly or in combination, make it difficult for sufferers to maintain an active role in the labour force include the following. First, dyspnoea and energy loss, resulting in a limited capacity for ambulation, mobility and any sort of manual work. Second, recurrent bouts of chest infection causing frequent periods of sickness absence, particularly in the cold winter months. Third, the anxiety, depression and 'somatic pre-occupations' that frequently accompany COAD and further hamper 'a good work adjustment' (Petty and Nett 1984). For example, Rutter (1979), in an evaluation of a management programme for COAD patients, found that psychological variables were strong predictors of vocational adjustment and work record after management. In contrast, physiological factors had very limited predictive value. Fourth, the additional rigours and demands which medical regimens (i.e. oxygen therapy, nebulisers, etc.) may impose. Finally, the inability to work in dusty, smoky atmospheres, or to come into contact with (noxious) fumes of any sort. As Rubeck, writing about the plight of the male bronchitic, states:

The patient suffering from disabling bronchitis, if he is still working, is almost certainly anxious about his job. He may be a skilled man working under ideal conditions and own a car in which he can avoid public transport. But even so there is the pervasive fear of sudden attacks of breathlessness, of more and more winter sick leave, of not achieving his full pension, of missing that final promotion which would make all the difference to contented retirement. The ... bronchitic may already have had to change his job from the trade he learned in youth, or the heavy outdoor work he enjoyed, to something less skilled or less strenuous, less enjoyable, less well paid. The writing is on the wall and he knows it.

He becomes breathless on exertion, in bad weather, or as a result of emotional upset or aggravation. Even the frustration engendered by his physical limitations seems to make him short of breath, and he becomes inwardly miserable and outwardly irritable, especially at the end of the day, when he returns home exhausted, fit for nothing but his armchair. . . . When bronchitis becomes so disabling that a man loses his job, his search for suitable work is fraught with difficulties.

(1971: 20–1)

Meanwhile the Royal College of Physicians' (RCP) report on disabling chest disease states:

> The onset of disabling disease affects employment, particularly if the job is physically demanding, if there is exposure to fumes or if it involves climbing many stairs or much travelling by public transport. Initially the onset may be concealed, as other workers may protect disabled colleagues from arduous tasks. Subsequently, when the condition is recognised, disabled employees in large firms may be accommodated in suitable work. Small firms may be unable to afford such re-deployment and, as a result, their disabled employee has to search for more suitable work and, if unsuccessful, draw unemployment or sickness benefit. He may try job after job, frequently taking unsuitable work in an attempt to continue as the breadwinner of his family. Sooner or later he may settle for long-term invalidity benefit. The contrast between the diminishing number of hospital admissions for chronic bronchitis and the persistently large numbers receiving invalidity benefit suggests that many disabled people adopt this last course; the supposition is consistent with clinical experience, but needs to be further explored.
>
> (1981: 81)

Rubeck's reference to the situation as 'fraught' is indeed apposite. In a highly competitive economic climate, suitable alternative work is seldom available, even for the able-bodied, and is readily taken up by younger, fitter, members of the workforce. Sufferers may not be registered for work as disabled persons either because they know nothing of its advantages, dislike the idea, have fallen foul of it, or because their general practitioner, in view of the employment problems within the area, has signed them off as unemployable (Rubeck 1971). Indeed, COAD is a difficult condition to place due to winter absenteeism and morning slowness. Moreover, many are probably deemed too old and medically unsuitable for industrial rehabilitation or the various government re-training schemes available (RCP 1981). Consequently, as Rubeck concludes: 'There is thus very little encouragement for the severely disabled bronchitic who still struggles to earn his living' (1971: 22). Whereas, concerning the results of her own study, she states:

> It has been noticeable in this study that most men, especially the middle-aged whose bronchitis prevents them from following their normal occupation, tend to accept permanent unemployment as the only alternative somewhat readily, and it is not difficult to see why. If

his doctor concurs with this negative outlook, the unemployed bronchitic will soon begin to regard himself as on the scrap heap for good.

(1971: 22)

Yet the extent of occupational disadvantage is not necessarily a direct function of the degree of impairment or disability experienced. Rather:

the kinds of problems chronically sick and disabled people encounter at work depend upon the nature of the disorder from which they suffer, the nature of the task they are called upon to do and the nature of the physical and social environment in which they work. Some of these problems are related to the specific work task itself; others are identical to more general practical problems of daily living. The extent to which the problems can be managed or solved determines whether or not the person concerned is able to remain at work. This may demand the job be restructured to suit a person with reduced capabilities, that the environment be modified to remove physical barriers to effective performance, or it may require the assistance and co-operation of colleagues and those in authority.

(Locker 1983: 99)

Indeed, COAD tends to create far greater problems for those in manual *vis-à-vis* non-manual occupations. The highly skewed social class distribution of the condition serves to exacerbate these tendencies. This is not, of course, to suggest that non-manual occupations are wholly unproblematic. Rather, that the magnitude and scale of occupational problems experienced by manual workers in the face of COAD generally tends to be greater, whilst their ability to be solved, and indeed the degree of scope and flexibility in resolving them, tends to be correspondingly smaller. In particular, given comparable levels of disability, those in non-manual occupations may be able to continue working far longer than their manual counterparts.

Occupational problems were commonly experienced by those in Williams' (1990) study. Indeed, as Table 4.1 showed, the work category of the FLP yielded the highest profile score of all twelve areas covered (42 per cent), men tending to score higher than women in this domain (p <.03). Forty per cent were unable to work owing to their illness, whilst 50 per cent of those who were now retired had previously been unable to work as a consequence of their illness. Many spoke of the struggle, difficulties and problems they experienced either currently or in the past prior to finishing work. Mr Bush, for example, a painter and decorator by trade, graphically described the problems he faced:

Well it became increasingly difficult for me to do me job, you know, hold it down, keep me head above water like. For a start it was increasingly difficult just getting to work on time in the mornings, and then there was the job itself. Looking back now I suppose I was pushing myself beyond my limits, you know, until one morning, I got as far as the corner of the road and I had to turn back, I nearly collapsed I was so breathless.

I mean I used to be up at 3 in the morning worrying over me work. You see I had it in me mind that if I didn't work I couldn't survive. If I didn't work, how could I manage? The writing was on the wall and I suppose I knew it. But, as I say, apart from the fact of having to get up earlier in the mornings, there was the problem of actually doing the job. I kept falling behind with me work, I couldn't keep up the pace. Fortunately, I worked on me own. I was given a specified time for each place and then a supervisor would come round once a day and check how I was gettin' on like, you know, which was a continual source of worry to me 'cause I was slowing down all the time. And I mean the job involved going up and down ladders and moving about, constantly moving about, reaching, bending and stretching and what have you, and in the end I just couldn't manage it. Besides the paint was doing me chest no good. I used to keep me inhalers in me pocket and have to keep stopping for a rest and a puff like, you know. Looking back I don't know how I did it, I didn't really realise how ill I was, or at least I didn't want to admit it. I just wanted to be 'normal' and kept hoping against hope that things would improve.

Similarly Mr Doyal, who had been a window cleaner for some twenty years, also found his job increasingly difficult to manage as his illness progressed. He claimed that he used to get very breathless because of the sheer physical exertion involved in his job, particularly climbing up and down ladders. Thus as time went on he noticed himself becoming less and less productive, describing his experience at work as one of 'puffing and bluffing'. Finally, following various unsuccessful attempts at finding suitable alternative work, he had to concede defeat and finish work altogether. However, he still clung on to the vain hope that one day he might be able to return to work, although he knew that in reality this was unlikely. In contrast, Mr Pinter was forced to finish work when he developed 'bronchial asthma' owing to his continual contact with flour as a baker in a top London hotel, later officially acknowledged as an industrial accident. As he put it: 'The heat, the steam, the flour, and all the running around the job involved, all them "ingredients" was a disaster for me in my condition.'

However, as mentioned earlier, whilst those in non-manual occupations tend to experience less severe and less intractable employment problems – enabling them to continue work considerably longer than their manual counterparts – such jobs are not without their own distinctive set of problems and difficulties. Mr Thompson, for example, a former college lecturer, described both positive and negative aspects of his job:

Well, you know, for instance, if the lifts were out of action, I couldn't get up the stairs, or walking from classroom to classroom, you know, some days that would give me terrible problems. I used to travel up by car because I had my own little parking space so, you know, that helped me because, again, I would probably have had to have given up work long before that if I hadn't been able to drive. And ah, of course, I was fortunate having the sort of job I had. I mean I only used to have to be in college four days a week, because I used to work two evenings a week and have Fridays off you see. The college was open 9.00 am till 9.00 pm, so I could span my work over quite a long day, which meant I could do most of the things I wanted or needed to do at a leisurely pace. Had I been doing something physical, I would have probably had to have packed up work much sooner, but I was able to go on for quite a long while like that. And of course, we used to get very long holidays, and you sort of get regular breaks. So basically my job really suited my problem.

But towards the end I was getting quite breathless and it was getting difficult, you know, at work really. Fortunately, the job I had did consist largely of administration. Also I was in charge of time-tabling and things like that, so I was able to select what I wanted to do to a large extent in my work and that too enabled me to keep at work much longer than I could otherwise have done. I was in a very privileged position. And also towards the end I was having to have quite a lot of time off work. Well it wasn't time off so much as the fact that in the winter when you get these bugs, they're very hard to shake off, you don't really ever get them right and you're always working under a bit of duress. You've either got to say to them 'All right', I mean, if I'd have said to my GP 'Oh I don't feel up to it' he'd have probably just kept putting me off sick, but you can't spend all your time being sick, you know. So once the old antibiotics had got a hold on things and I felt a bit better I used to go back to work didn't I [to his wife]? If it hadn't been for the way I fiddled my own timetable I'd have had a lot more time off. And in the end I was sort of having time off, time off, and, ah, it was also getting increasingly difficult in the winter. I mean, I'd sort of clean the old blackboard after a lecture and I'd have to sort of sit down for ten minutes to catch my breath back. And I was running out of breath when I taught, I didn't seem to have enough wind to talk properly and at length even then.

Other commonly voiced problems included the difficulties involved in actually getting to work on time in the mornings; the problems involved in commuting to and from work on public transport, especially in the cold, wet winter months; the sheer effort involved in trying to maintain and hold down a regular job when ill; the erratic pattern of sickness absence; trying to avoid having too much time off work; problems of attempting to 'keep up' and 'cover up' at work; and, finally, feeling tired and worn out at the end of the day and having precious little energy left to do anything else.

The 'limits of tolerance' of employers, colleagues and workmates

What has been said so far relates only to the problems and difficulties COAD sufferers face in carrying out the actual tasks, duties and responsibilities of their occupation roles. Yet vocational roles are not, of course, carried out in isolation from one another. Rather, they necessitate having to work with and for others within an increasingly complex and specialised division of labour. Yet as Bury (1982, 1988) suggests, we know relatively little about the 'limits of tolerance' regarding family, friends, workmates and colleagues and how these vary according to differing social settings, circumstances and socio-economic backgrounds.

A number of those in Williams' (1990) study, for example, spoke of how workmates had helped 'carry' them, help them out, or 'cover' for them when off sick. For instance, Mr Brown, who had worked in the distribution and despatch department of a leading national newspaper, spoke of how his friends and colleagues had helped carry him. As he put it: 'They were a good bunch . . . I didn't have to lift a finger in the end.' Mr Wilkinson, a stationery storeman, also spoke of how his colleagues would lend a hand with the deliveries, whilst Mr Ash, a chauffeur for a national shipping company, spoke of how friends and colleagues, many of whom 'owed me a few favours', would help load and unload the luggage in the car and carry it aboard the ship for him when he arrived at his destination. However, for Mr Ash, as for many others, this situation was wholly unacceptable, adding a further dimension of pressure, a moral imperative, upon him to finish work altogether despite claiming to love his job. In this respect, the weight of social credits appeared to have reached what was deemed to be an unacceptable and intolerable level. As he put it:

It was becoming increasingly difficult. I mean, lots of people started helping to do me job for me, I mean lots of different jobs. For example, I'd say 'Oh can you tell so and so for me' instead of me having to go aboard ship and tell them myself, or 'Oh, can you bring this case up or down for me', 'cause I couldn't do it myself, so they used to do it. So in the end I was having to ask other people to do all the rushing around for me, you know, relying on their good-will, the good-will that I'd accrued over the years I suppose. I could drive from A to B, but when I got out of the car, well I couldn't do it, I was having to rely on others to help me out and that was unacceptable to me. If I couldn't do the job properly I shouldn't be doing it at all, that's the way I felt.

Others, however, had not been so fortunate. Miss Bell, for example, spoke of her employers' general lack of understanding and tolerance regarding her illness and her time off work:

Oh they [employers] weren't very supportive. A few times when I was off sick, they'd send a letter saying that they would have to employ somebody else if I couldn't give them a definite date of return. And I would phone them up and say: 'Put yourself in my shoes, how can I give you a definite date? If I was feeling well I'm sure I would be there.' And I'd have to get my doctor to write a letter saying I was all right to work in a canteen and that I would be back as soon as possible. But the bosses at work, they weren't very considerate, not very helpful and supportive. I feel they could have done more, been a bit more tolerant and understanding, you know, made life a bit easier for me.

Mr Porter, who still worked in the upholstery trade, also seemed very uncertain of the 'limits of tolerance' of both his employer and colleagues towards his illness; hence he strategically played down his chest trouble at work. Indeed, he seemed to have adopted a pragmatic non-disclosure policy at work; one very similar to that which Scambler (1989) describes in his study of epileptics. In his mind, it seemed a very real possibility that the implication of disclosure might in some way jeopardise his job either currently or in the future. Finally, those who were self-employed and worked single-handedly (e.g. freelance carpenters, painters and decorators, etc.) faced the double jeopardy of not only forgone earnings, but also a potential loss of trade in the future through obtaining a reputation of 'unreliabilty'.

Occupational drift

In her study of the lives of 194 people disabled by a variety of conditions, Blaxter (1976) found two predominant occupational career patterns: 'discontinuity' and 'drift'. The former involved a fairly rapid and abrupt transition from work to unemployment, whilst the latter involved a slow drift down the occupational scale through a series of less well paid, less satisfying and less rewarding work, until finally drifting into a similar position of unemployment. Also Meadows (1961), in an earlier disease-specific study of the occupational careers of middle-aged chronic bronchitics, found a marked concentration of patients in social class V during the previous decade when compared to a control group. Consequently, she concluded that the class gradient in mortality from chronic bronchitis could at least partly be explained by health-related downward social mobility. However, caution is needed in interpreting Meadows' findings, as her sample consisted of hospitalised chronic bronchitics and may, therefore, be unrepresentative, identifying the particular type of bronchitics who are hospitalised rather than highlighting downward social drift as such (Blane 1985). Moreover, Meadows' study also took place in a period when employment patterns and job opportunities were very different from today.

In Williams' (1990) more recent study of COAD, for example, only 14 per cent of those who were currently working or who had worked in their lives claimed to have experienced downward social mobility as a consequence of their illness – some of these, in fact, actually involved movement *within* rather than between the Registrar General's occupational classes. Indeed, in the present economic climate, withdrawal from the labour market seems a far more likely option than a change of job for those who suffer from COAD. As mentioned earlier, once COAD has reached a certain stage of development it is unlikely that the individual can ever work again, whilst many of the jobs on offer to people with disabilities appear quite unsuitable for those suffering from chronic respiratory illness and disability (RCP 1981).

A good example of occupational 'drift', however, concerned the case of Mr Kerr. A painter and decorator by trade, he was forced to finish work when his illness became worse. He then spent approximately a year out of work before obtaining a job as a cleaner – a job which appeared most unsuitable, although he claimed the work was 'light'. He managed to struggle on for another couple of years doing this job until:

> I had a bad turn, I got a lot of acid fumes one morning off the cleaning

fluids, I took it all in . . . and I got a bad fit of coughing . . . just couldn't stop, I just couldn't, so they sent me home.

After this he never returned to work again. Similarly, Mr Watson had had to change from his trade as bricklayer to that of care-taker, whilst Mr Doyal had left his job of some twenty years as a window cleaner, which he claimed was 'well paid', and switched to what he thought would be 'lighter work' as a canteen assistant on a building site. This, he claimed, involved a considerable drop in pay and after a short time also proved unsuitable and beyond him. Bereft as to what to do, he went back to window cleaning, being assigned an indoor job at a top London hotel which he described as 'lighter, easier work'. Finally, when he found that this too was beyond him, he drifted into unemployment.

However, the predominant pattern in Williams' (1990) study was one of remaining and struggling on in the same occupation until, eventually, it became too much and then either having to finish work altogether or take early retirement. Some, however, actually managed to struggle on and make it to normal retirement age. It was also notable how the pattern of early retirement, or of finishing work at official state retirement age, tended to favour those in non-manual *vis-à-vis* manual occupations, as one may perhaps expect. Thus Mr Thompson (a college lecturer) and Mr Richardson (a technical adviser), for example, not only were able to continue in their jobs far longer than would otherwise have been the case in manual occupations, but also were able to take early retirement on very favourable terms. Similarly, Mr Kepple, a managing director of his own company, despite being considerably disabled, managed to work right up to, and indeed past, official state retirement age, owing to both the nature of his job and the high degree of flexibility and autonomy he enjoyed.

Disadvantage in the labour market

Not only does chronic illness and disability create problems whilst at work, it also creates disadvantage in the labour market for those who are without work, but who are still actively seeking it. As we have seen, whilst it is unlikely once COAD has reached a certain stage of development that the sufferer will ever work again, those who still seek work may experience considerable disadvantage in the labour market as a consequence of their illness and disability. Miss Bell, for example, after a considerable struggle in the face of her progressively worsening condition, was made redundant. Worried about what she was going to do with 'a flat to keep and no job, I went spare'; she searched desperately and unsuccessfully for six months for another job. However, as she stated, whenever she went for interviews, 'they'd say "Oh, do you suffer with your breathing?", or "Are you asthmatic?" And then they'd say "Oh well", you know, "we'll let you know" sort of thing.' Eventually her consultant, on discovering the anxious state she was getting herself in over her employment situation, and in view of her worsening illness, signed her off as permanently unfit for work.

Another example concerned the case of Mr Wilkinson, who had been made redundant from his previous post as stationery storeman and was unemployed for some time. He actively, yet unsuccessfully, sought work before finally realising the impossibility of the situation, and was then transferred onto long-term invalidity benefit. As he put it:

> Well after being made redundant I signed on the labour and I kept me eyes peeled for anything suitable that might come up, you know, I thought to myself 'Well if something comes up', but I couldn't find anything. And then this postal messinger job come up. Anyway I went up there and it was too much walkin' around in the City and no way could I have done it, there was too much walkin' about . . . and so I had to let that go. I knew what me capabilities was. And besides, it was the firm I'd originally started with. . . . And being what a good record I had, I wouldn't have wanted to take the job on knowing I couldn't do it, you know, and so I had to let it go. I didn't want to risk a good reputation on something I knew I wouldn't be able to do like, you know.
>
> Anyway, after that things became progressively worse, to the extent that I cannot work at all now, that's it. I know there ain't no chance of me finding any work now, 'cause I mean, let's face it, if you can't walk anywhere and you keep on getting out of breath when you try to do anything, you know, you can't lift and what have you, then who's gonna employ you? There ain't much chance of finding work then is there. I mean, it's hard enough when you're fit and healthy these days in't it, so what chance would I have. Besides, physically I don't feel up to it any more, my workin' days are over.

Similarly, Mr Pinter, after having to finish work as a baker in a top London hotel owing to his illness, also became unemployed. Despite attempts to find suitable alternative work – for example, he attempted to re-train in a government Employment Rehabilitation Centre as a clock and watch repairer, but, as the RCP (1981) report discusses, found that the spirits used to clean the mechanisms and the general atmosphere of the workshop affected his chest – he too was unsuccessful.

Of course, chronic illness and disability affects not only the lives of sufferers themselves, but also those of their families and kinsfolk. Thus wives may be forced to give up their jobs in order to care for their sick husbands or, perhaps less frequently, vice versa. For example, Mr Boyle, a devoted husband, had given up his job as steward of a social club in order to care for his severely disabled wife, whilst Mrs Kerr had also given up her part-time job as a cleaner as it was 'all getting too much' for her. As she stated:

> Oh I think that, oh I got a bit depressed and I think it all got too much for me, you know . . . I wasn't getting any rest see, because I had to keep getting up for my husband and, umh, I wasn't having enough rest, it all got too much. Well, by the end of it I was really exhausted, worn out, you know. Then I went to my doctor and he said 'Oh give the job up' and so I packed it up . . . I mean, I was getting so tired that come dinner time, you know, I felt I wanted to cry.

Mrs Bush was also in a similar position, having had to finish work fairly recently. As she explained:

> Well I used to have a part-time cleaning job, and I mean it used to get me out of the house and bring in a bit of extra money each week like, you know, help supplement the income a bit. But I had to give it up 'cause it was all becoming too much for me, I was exhausted and, besides, I couldn't leave him on his own. I mean, it's so unpredictable these days that you're scared to leave him, there's no warning like, it comes on so sudden. So I had to give it up.

However, faced with severe financial hardship, some may be forced to continue to work, despite wishing to care for their sick spouse at home. Mrs Charlton, for example, was forced by their precarious financial circumstances to continue working full-time, now being the sole breadwinner in the household. Yet she also spoke of how she wished to be at home in order to care for her husband – claiming that she did not like leaving him on his own all day long. Moreover, she appeared uncertain as to her entitlements regarding state benefits. Thus she continued to work full-time, yet worried considerably about her husband's welfare.

THE MEANING AND SYMBOLIC SIGNIFICANCE OF WORK

The ability to perform the various tasks, activities and roles which together constitute an individual's daily life and social world has implications at both the practical and symbolic levels: what Bury (1988) has appositely termed meaning as *consequence* and meaning as *significance*. In this respect vocational roles are often a major source of value and identity. Consequently, the loss of work, coupled with the knowledge of one's inability ever to work again, may have profound implications for the individual at both the practical and symbolic levels.

Agle *et al.* (1973), for example, found that if patients were able to work, their self-esteem increased and depression lessened. Perhaps not surprisingly, depression increased if the patient learned he or she could not continue to work and employment was a highly prized and valued role. Similarly, many of those in Williams' (1990) study, regardless of their occupation, spoke of the profound moral, social, psychological and symbolic impact which the loss of work had had upon them, and also of the (retrospective) meaning and significance which work assumed. Mr Thomas, for example, graphically explained the circumstances surrounding having to finish work and of his feelings regarding this:

> Well I had to go in as an in-patient in January '86 and they kept me in for three or four weeks. And when I came out I was still too ill to return to work. Anyway, next time I attended my out-patient appointment in the February of that year, they kept me in again. And this time [Dr R] said to me: 'Well Mr Thomas, I'm sorry to say that you're going to have to finish work, your working days are over.' And I looked at him and I said: 'You're bleedin' joking aren't you, tell me you're joking', and he said: 'No, I'm sorry but I'm not'. . . . And then he told me that I would have to go on oxygen, that they would be getting an oxygen machine installed at home for me, and that I'd have to stay on it for 16 hours a day. And the other doctor [Dr W], he said: 'And we must emphasise 16 hours a day', and they wouldn't let me go home until they had installed it. Honestly, one minute I thought I was going to be all right, and the next minute I'm told I'm never gonna work again and that I'm gonna have to be stuck on oxygen for 16 hours a bleedin' day!
>
> It was quite a . . . shock then to be honest with you. I felt as if my world was crumbling about my ears. But then you still don't really believe it's happening to you at the time, it doesn't really sink in until later when you've got time to reflect on it like. It all seemed to happen so fast: Bang!

He continued, regarding the value of work and his feelings at not being able to work any more:

> Well it's frustrating, 'cause it is, it's frustrating not being able to work. Frustrating, boring, less money, any which way you wanna look at it really, it's all them things. 'Cause you can't do anything without work as far as I'm concerned. Really I feel gutted, that I've lost out, you know what I mean. And I mean I miss it, I do. And seeing me workmates every day, having a chat, you know, the company like. I mean I'd love to be able to get up one morning and go off to work. Yeah, I miss it.

Whereas, concerning its impact on his self-image and sense of identity, he stated:

> You feel out of the main stream of society, a reject, bleedin' useless, on the scrap heap, can't do nothing. 'Cause you're not pulling your weight, you're not doing nothing in society are you, you're dependent on others all the time; the state, your family. You lose your independence and your self-respect. I mean, I know I'm not totally dependent on others, but we're [his wife was disabled too] well on the way to being so.

The inability to work may bring in its wake, particularly in the early stages before 'resignation' sets in, a sense of there being a tremendous void or gulf in one's life which is difficult to fill. In particular, the loss of a sense of structure, order, meaning and purpose in daily life may occur. Consequently feelings of boredom may result, with suitable and satisfactory alternatives to work being at best hard to find and at worst non-existent. As Mr O'Riley remarked:

> Well there's nothing to do but look at that [TV] . . . [and] . . . of late it seems to be gettin' to me. Before it wasn't, but just lately it seems to be gettin' to me a bit more. Some days it drives you crackers. I mean, there's not a lot you can do now, and there's not a lot you can do about it. And, ah, well as I say, it does get to you after a while, you know. I mean I must admit I get very frustrated and depressed about it at times, you know, and then I tend to get a bit short tempered.

In essence, the meaning and symbolic significance of work for the chronically sick and disabled revolves around three main factors: first, the intrinsic satisfaction which work itself may provide, together with the sense of routine and order it brings to daily life; second, the loss of economic and financial independence and the concomitant feelings of dependency, of 'being useless', and a 'drain on society' which having to finish work may engender; finally, the often intense feelings of frustration, depression, boredom and monotony which may arise as a consequence of having to finish work, together with the loss of social contact and company which work provides.

PROBLEMS OF INCOME

Another all too frequent and unfortunate consequence of chronic illness and disability, particularly for those who have to finish work, concerns the creation of varying degrees of financial hardship. The relationship, however, is not necessarily linear in nature. Rather, it is influenced by many other intervening factors; perhaps the main one being occupational and socio-economic status. Generally, however, and unfortunately all too often, chronic illness and disability results, in the long run, in a reduced income and hence a decline in living standards. As Locker notes:

> The loss of physical resources that stems from chronic disease almost invariably leads to a loss of material resources in the form of money and wealth. It should come as no surprise then to find that all studies of long-term sickness or poverty have found a correlation between the two. It could be argued that disabled people who receive a low income are more disadvantaged than the able-bodied poor if only because disability creates extra needs and entails extra expense. . . . Consequently, a limited income has to be spread that much further. For example, the disabled need to spend more on heating, special clothing, and diets, or they may need to replace clothing and furniture more frequently because of damage caused by wheelchairs and other aids. . . . Perhaps a more important source of disadvantage is this: the reduced financial resources at the disposal of disabled people need to be spent in ways which compensate for their reduced capacity to perform the mundane practical tasks of everyday life. . . . It is lack of money as much as the illness and its effects which prevents them from pursuing and attaining the good things in life.
>
> (1983: 119–20)

As Locker's quote suggests, many studies have pointed to the relationship between chronic illness and financial and material disadvantage (Blaxter 1976, Townsend 1979, West 1989). Perhaps the most important and most recent of these, however, concerns the OPCS report on 'The financial circumstances of disabled adults living in private households' (OPCS 1988b). As the report states:

The survey shows two broad effects of disability on the financial circumstances of disabled adults. As a consequence of being less likely than the population as a whole to have earned income disabled adults have on average lower incomes than the rest of the population: disabled adults are both less likely to work and, if they are able to work, likely to earn less than adults in general. . . . The majority of disabled adults incur extra expenditure as a consequence of being disabled, the amount of which is related to the nature and severity of their disability, and also to the income they have available to spend in connection with their disability. Overall, disabled adults are likely to experience some financial problems and to have lower standards of living than the population as a whole as a result of having lower average incomes.

(1988b: xviii)

As mentioned above, although all forms of chronic illness and disability tend to create additional financial problems and difficulties, the demands particular conditions place on sufferers' lives create their own *specific* pattern of financial problems and difficulties. Scarce resources have to be strategically and selectively allocated in order to compensate for, and attempt to overcome, the specific challenges, problems and difficulties by the illness and the specific character, nature and severity of the associated disability. Thus musculo-skeletal conditions may create different financial challenges to those of, say, a respiratory nature. These in turn may differ in kind from those created by various chronic neurological and psychiatric disorders. Hence, it is to a discussion of such issues in relation to COAD that this chapter now turns.

Living and managing on a reduced income

It can be readily appreciated how varying degrees of financial disadvantage – ranging from extreme financial hardship to a marginal loss of income and decline in living standards – all too often accompany the arrival of a chronic, disabling condition. For example, as Nocon and Booth (1991) found in their recent study of the social impact of asthma, the condition 'often had an impact on respondents' finances'. Common problems were the loss of income due to sufferers or their families either having to finish or take time off work due to the illness. Extra costs associated with asthma (i.e. one-off purchases such as non-allergenic bedding or more regular expenses such as prescriptions or additional heating) were also often mentioned. Indeed, a number of respondents in their study felt that some of the problems caused by their asthma might be alleviated if they had more money; enabling them, for example, to purchase a nebuliser.

It is also clear that the consequences of chronic illness and disability are 'socially patterned' (MacIntyre 1986, 1988) in terms of socio-economic status and a variety of other indicators of inequality. As we have seen, not only does COAD interfere considerably with the sufferer's ability to work, but also the fact that it disproportionately affects those from manual working-class backgrounds means that the financial disadvantage it brings in its wake may be considerable. Moreover, several studies have demonstrated the link between economic security and general life satisfaction. Young (1982), for example, in a study of COAD patients and their spouses, found that patients' monetary resources, in addition to their personal resources (i.e. positive illness perceptions, knowledge of the illness, regimen compliance, etc.), predicted better adaptation. Also, wives of COAD patients in Sexton and Monro's (1985) study reported greater satisfaction with life if they were satisfied with their financial circumstances.

A drop in income and financial problems and difficulties were also commonly experienced by those in Williams' (1990) study. Seventeen per cent stated that they were currently experiencing 'moderate financial problems and difficulties' due to their illness, whilst a further 25 per cent admitted to 'marked problems and difficulties' – the remainder (58 per cent) experiencing 'no' or only 'slight problems and difficulties'. Statistically significant differences were also found between social class and financial problems and difficulties, with manual workers (Registrar General's social classes IIIM, IV and V) tending to experience financial problems and difficulties of a moderate or marked nature far more frequently than their non-manual (Registrar General's social classes I, II and IIINM) counterparts (p <.01).

As these figures suggest, the scope, range and nature of financial problems and difficulties experienced may vary considerably, particularly in relation to social class. Thus, although all of those in Williams' (1990) study who had finished work through illness had taken a drop in income, some were more fortunate than others. For example, Mr Thompson, who had been able to take early retirement from his post as a lecturer at a technical college, spoke of how this had created very little in the way of financial problems and difficulties. He claimed that he had anticipated just such a happening; thus he had been able to plan ahead and make financial provisions for a reasonably 'secure and comfortable future'. As he put it:

No, once again you see, it was something that I knew was coming and so we had begun to make certain provisions for it hadn't we [to his wife]? . . . I mean we live quite well and, you know, we can afford to live reasonably well, and we haven't got any great yearnings for anything really. . . . So I haven't really got any fears and worries about financial security, I'm quite fortunate in that respect I suppose.

Some, in contrast, were in a *transitional* state: whilst things were 'not too bad' at the moment, the future seemed much more problematic, bleak and uncertain. For example, Mr Thomas was, at the time of interview, managing to keep his 'head above water'. However, he expressed considerable worry financially over his future when his company sickness benefit scheme – paid for a maximum of two years – ran out, his savings dwindled, and he was left to rely solely on the 'tender mercies' of the state. As he put it:

Well, at first I thought things were going to be all right. But now I can foresee what's going to happen: as time goes on things are going to become increasingly tighter and tighter, especially when me [company] sick pay runs out. I mean it's already beginning to bite, me savings are gradually dwindling. I mean, you can't buy what you want, when you want, you have to be more careful now, cut down on things. Things that once you would have gone out and bought, things that once you would have replaced, you have to make do with now.

Others, however, unfortunately were already in 'dire financial straits'. Mr Pinter, for instance, whose wife was also disabled and who had a young daughter to support, described his financial position as 'a disaster' since finishing work. This appeared to be no exaggeration. Indeed, he claimed that one of the biggest problems concerning his illness was the financial hardship it had created. As he stated:

You name it, we've had to cut down on it or do without. There's lots of things we can't afford and we have to go without now. I mean there's the telephone, can't afford no telephone. No car. And then there's things for these two, my daughter and my wife, you know clothes and what have you, you know what the youngsters are today, they want this and they want that 'cause their friends have got it.

   By the time we've paid the rent and the electric and for our food, it does not leave a lot spare for anything else, it does not. I mean, talking about clothes, I've gotta pair of trousers, some old'uns, you know with bell bottoms, I've had 'em altered to straighten them out, and I've still got the suit I was married in, I'm still wearing it! It's like I want to buy a pair of shoes and it's a sore point at the moment, 'cause I've gotta find enough money to buy some shoes for meself. And I mean, I'd like to buy another televison but I cannot afford it.

Similarly, Miss Bell, who lived alone, was also in a precarious position. It was clear that she experienced considerable financial worry, difficulty and hardship. As she stated:

Oh, I've had to cut lots of 'luxuries' out now. I have to think twice about spending money on anything now. I've either had to cut down on or do without everything from fruit and fruit juice to clothes and things for the home; everything other than the basics. I mean your food, heating and the telephone – I must have the telephone, it's a life-line for me see – it's all gotta come out of that little bit of money. And it worries me 'cause I think to meself: 'Will I have enough, am I always going to make ends meet?'

Mr Charlton, meanwhile, tellingly remarked:

Money, that's the major problem . . . the problems with the illness you could get over to a certain extent, or at least cope with better, if you had enough money couldn't you? You ain't got that worry on your plate have you? If you've got worry on your plate, worry over money and how you're gonna live next week, what you've got to live on next week, it's definitely gonna fetch things on what it shouldn't. If you've got no worry, then it's gotta be easier ain't it? . . . I mean you ain't gotta worry about next week have you? Or I'm looking at a pair of shoes, I need a new pair of shoes, 'Oh I can't afford a pair of shoes', you understand what I mean.

Yet despite, or rather in the face of, these financial problems and difficulties, the chronically sick and disabled have little choice but to attempt to manage on what they have. Thus in addition to 'cutting-down' and 'doing without', other strategies such as the careful budgeting, management and selective allocation of limited income may have to be devised. Such strategies frequently involve juggling, balancing and trading-off competing needs and priorities against one another; the end result being that one just 'manages to get by'. A policy in which self-restraint, a tightening of one's belt, and a rigorous avoidance or denial of all forms of financial 'self-indulgence' is required in order to 'get by' and avoid getting into debt. Miss Bell, for example, described how she carefully managed and budgeted her money and of how she rigorously avoided getting into debt:

Oh I'm very careful with my money, it's very carefully organised. I mean, I've never been a one to get into debt or have anything on the 'weekly'. When I get my money I divide it up and I put away for everything. Then, what's left is mine to spend and when it's gone it's gone.

Similarly, Mr Doyal remarked:

Well, what with the supplementary and what have you, I've adjusted meself, course I've had to tighten me belt, but as I say, I've adjusted meself . . . I have to set aside so much a week for each thing like. But by the time I've paid for me shopping, me heating, me washing and I've put a bit away for the telephone, I haven't got a lot left over each week, there's nothing left over, you know. But then again I don't go out anywhere so, you know, and I am careful with what I have coming in each week. So I manage to get by just about, it just ekes out, whatever I get, it just about ekes out right, you know.

These accounts illustrate two things. First, that in the face of financial hardship, sufferers and their families 'manage to get by' via a range of strategies, self-denials and stringent budgetary controls, and, second, that the very concept of 'managing to get by' may conceal as much as it reveals – covering a broad range of experience from minor to severe financial hardship and disadvantage.

Additional expenses

Perhaps one of the most frequently cited sources of additional expenditure in relation to chronic respiratory illness concerns the increased heating costs incurred in the cold winter months. Many of those in Williams' (1990) study, for example, spoke of how their heating bills had increased, sometimes dramatically, since the illness – partly as a consequence of being at home all day, and partly due to the illness directly and the necessity of keeping warm. Moreover, this was further compounded by the fact that many of their homes were not double-glazed or centrally heated and consequently were difficult to heat and keep warm in the cold winter months. As Mrs Andrews put it concerning the additional expenses she incurred:

Oh yeah, well there's the heating. I find I use a lot of heat in the winter, 'cause I can't be cold. 'Cause if I get cold then that's when it starts me coughing, you know, when the atmosphere gets very cold and damp, and then I'm prone to chest infections see. So I have to keep meself warm, and the heating bills are high in the winter, 'cause it's a very cold place here . . . I mean that's a major bill.

Others also spoke of how the general cost of everything in the home had risen as a consequence of being at home all day. As Mr Thomas stated:

Also, of course, there's the general point that all your expenses go up, from food and heating bills right through to toilet rolls, especially with us both being ill, 'cause you're at home all the time. So in that sense we're actually spending more nowadays.

Other sources of additional expenditure may, of course, include transportation costs and the attempt to remain mobile, prescription charges, aids and appliances (if not free), additional clothing, the costs of having to pay others to do things such as painting, decorating, household maintenance and repair work and so on (Walker 1981).

Mr O'Riley, for example, claimed that public transport was beyond him nowadays and had to rely on taxis or the good will of others. However, having only a limited income to live on, he found taxi fares very expensive and hard to afford; thus he had to limit taxi rides to essential journeys. Consequently, in the absence of a mobility allowance – for which he was in the process of appealing for the third time – he claimed that he was prohibited from maintaining and enjoying a greater degree of mobility in and around the community which such an allowance would help facilitate. Indeed, perhaps one of the major bones of contention regarding welfare benefits to emerge within Williams' (1990) study, concerned the issue of eligibility for mobility allowance. As Hunter (1986) has shown, an analysis of a sample of recipients of mobility allowance revealed them to be a quite heterogeneous group in relation to the degree of disability they experienced. Moreover, the eligibility criteria adopted for this allowance – subsumed from April 1992 under the new Disability Living Allowance – tend to be geared more towards musculo-skeletal types of disability and 'traditional' ADL items; hence they tend to discriminate against those 'worthy' applicants who suffer from respiratory illness and disability (Williams 1989b).

There were many examples of candidates whose disability and circumstances clearly warranted the awarding of a mobility allowance, and who would have benefited considerably from it, but who had either been turned down, or were currently appealing (sometimes for a third time) against what they felt to be an 'unfair' and 'unjust' decision. For example, Mrs Cole remarked:

He [Doctor] examined my chest and made me walk a little bit, umh, up the stairs and such like. And then I got a letter sayin', ah it said on it something like, 'Because you are not physically disabled enough, blah, blah, blah . . .', you know, it's like I said to you, you gotta be in a wheelchair or have a leg off before you get any of these things . . .

Well I was talkin' to a lady at the hospital Monday and she got it. And you have to end up, she says to me, 'Bleedin' lying to 'em' before, you know, not because you don't deserve or need it like, it's not that. In the end she said 'You have to end up lying to 'em', because they, you know. Looking back now, perhaps I was too honest, see I've never asked, I've never asked for anything. Me husband's always worked, I've always worked, and I've never been a one to, you know what I mean . . . again, I feel it reflects a lack of understanding in society-at-large, 'cause their standards, criteria or whatever, are geared to people with other types of disabilities aren't they? I mean a man in a wheelchair might not be able to walk across a room and so he's entitled to the mobility, but just because I can doesn't mean that I don't have difficulty gettin' about, that it ain't hard for me, 'cause I do and it is. So it tends to be geared to people like that, don't get me wrong, people like that are entitled to it, but so are many other people who don't get it, 'cause they don't fit into the right pigeon hole, it's ludicrous really.

This chapter has attempted to portray something of the broad range of occupational and financial disadvantage which COAD sufferers and their families may experience as a consequence of the illness. Many of these problems and difficulties are, of course, similar in kind to those experienced by the chronically sick and disabled populace as a whole. Others, however, stem from the specific nature of COAD as a disabling condition. Moreover, as we have seen, the nature and severity of the occupational problems and financial difficulties experienced differ not only according to the severity of COAD and the level of disability experienced, but also in relation to the socio-economic background of the sufferer. In this respect, the fact that COAD disproportionately affects those from a working-class background adds a further dimension of disadvantage to both sufferers and their families.

Chapter 6

Social and family life

As Charmaz (1983) suggests, it is the social aspects of chronic illness and disability and how they impinge upon self and others which are perhaps the most difficult to bear, adjust to and cope with. Similarly, in her study of the meaning of disability, Blaxter notes:

> Although the practical problems of work, money, and daily living seemed to be most prominent amongst the patients of this survey, it was social problems – family relationships, isolation and loneliness, lack of occupation and recreation – which were perhaps the most distressing.
>
> (1976: 218–19)

Hence, it is to a detailed discussion of such issues in relation to COAD that this chapter now turns.

SOCIAL LIFE, RECREATION AND PASTIMES

Social life

A common experience in the lives of the chronically sick and disabled concerns the decline of social life and its impact upon self-identity. As Charmaz states:

> Physical pain, psychological distress and the deleterious effects of medical procedures all cause the chronically ill to suffer as they experience their illness. However, a narrow medicalized view of suffering, solely defined as physical discomfort, ignores or minimizes the broader significance of the suffering experienced by debilitated chronically ill adults. A fundamental form of that suffering is the loss of self in chronically ill persons who observe their former self-images crumbling away without the simultaneous development of equally

valued new ones. As a result of their illness, these individuals suffer from (1) leading restricted lives, (2) experiencing social isolation, (3) being discredited and (4) burdening others.

(1983: 168)

In Williams' (1990) study, for example, the general picture was of COAD having had a considerable impact upon sufferers' social lives; of life appearing to become increasingly 'narrowed down' and restricted as the illness progressed (Bury 1978). Take, for example, the case of Mr O'Riley:

Mr O'Riley: Well, I've got no social life these days; non-existent I think is how you'd describe it. I get out and about very little these days, very little.

Interviewer: Would you attribute that to your illness?

Mr O'Riley: Well, I'd put it down to being as I can't get about very well, and the limitations and restrictions of the illness, where can I go like and what can I do?

Interviewer: Do you ever manage to go out and socialise?

Mr O'Riley: No. I can't even have a holiday or nothing 'cause, besides the illness, the way the money is it can't stretch that far. I'm just existing that's all, not living, just existing.

Similarly, Mr Thomas, who at one time had been the chairman of his local social club and had led a fairly full social life, stated:

Well, it's really non-existent these days. We don't see many people really do we [to wife], cut to the bone I s'pose you could say, gone up in a puff of smoke. We only go out to do the bare essentials really nowadays, plus sometimes maybe I'll have the occasional evening down at the local social club, you know, but she [wife] doesn't go though, not now.

Obviously, the underlying reasons for this dwindling of social life are many and varied. As Charmaz notes:

A major reason is that the ill person does not have adequate time, energy or concentration to sustain his or her relationships. Reorganizing priorities results in limited time. Because work comes first and exhausts those still able to manage it, they find they have no energy left for other involvements. In addition, simply managing daily maintenance takes longer when fatigue or discomfort is high, when energy is low and when medical procedures take time.

(1983: 177)

However, whilst such descriptions were fairly typical, most sufferers were still occupied in varying degrees with the struggle to maintain at least a semblance or vestige of their former social life – recognising its practical, psychological and symbolic importance. As Mr Bush put it, 'you need human contact don't you, otherwise you get stale, and then you begin to wilt and die inside'. Indeed many, despite the limitations of their illness and disability, strove to maintain their social life and their social contacts as best they could. Yet, set against the backdrop of the increasing physical limitations of the disease, the declining ability to maintain social contacts, and the withering of social support networks, this is not always an easy task.

Another important and salient theme contained within the accounts of Williams' (1990) respondents, concerned the problem of what Kelleher (1988), in his study of diabetes, terms the *loss of spontaneity*. Not only was the withering of social life frequently lamented, but reference was also often made to the way in which the illness denied patients and their families the ability to lead a normal, flexible, spontaneous and un-restricted social and recreational life. Very often, despite attempts to the contrary, it appeared that life was dominated or organised around the illness rather than vice versa. In particular, careful, often meticulous, arrangements and considerations may have to be made beforehand, regarding outings or social events. Activities, for instance, have to be carefully planned and made conditional upon how one feels on the day; the demands, problems and difficulties of medical regimens have to be considered and resolved; the perennial threat of picking up infections has to be carefully weighed; and the issue of whether or not other people smoke, or whether there will be a smoky atmosphere to contend with, also have to be taken into account. Unfortunately this, together with the sheer physical and mental effort involved in socialising and general feelings of embarrassment, may result in sufferers slowly withdrawing from social life; instead feeling more comfortable and secure in the privacy of their own homes.

Thus, concerning the 'loss of spontaneity' in her life, Mrs White, who was on long-term oxygen, stated: 'we can't just get in the car and go off like we used to be able to do, nothing's spontaneous any more, everything's got to be planned all the time'. Similarly, Mrs McLeod stated: 'it's the same with everything these days, whatever you want to do you've got to make arrangements for this, that and the other, it's such a palaver that sometimes you end up just not bothering in the end'. And Mr Brown remarked:

I have to plan everything so carefully these days, for instance; who I'm going to, where I'm going to, if the environment or the surroundings where I'm going are favourable or unfavourable, and whether, if I was visiting people, I could manage, or rather how long I could manage, to control my symptoms such as coughing and what have you. . . . Besides, both physically and mentally you just can't seem to get out as much as you used to, or as much as you'd like to, when you're like this: you just can't cope with people for too long. So of course it affects your social life, it must do.

Faced with such problems, the demise of social life in the wake of the illness may generate a profound sense of loss. As Mr O'Riley stated:

Oh I miss it, I miss it, very badly I miss it. I mean take going down to the pub, it's not that I used to drink, but it was the company, you know, you could wander down there of an evening or at the weekends, and have a few drinks with your mates, spend a couple of hours or so there, you know, and I miss that very badly. Nowadays there's nothing to do but look at that [television].

Moreover, it may also generate a sense of 'injustice' or 'unfairness' on the part of sufferers and their families concerning the illness and its curtailment of their lives. As Mr and Mrs Thomas remarked:

Mr Thomas: When I think that a few years ago me and Jerry at work were discussing retirement and that we was going to do, you know, 'When I'm 65' and all that sort of thing.

Mrs Thomas: Yes and when I was ill in hospital remember, you came in one evening and you said 'Never mind love, now we've got the kids off our hands we can enjoy ourselves', and what happened, he got ill didn't he, and now he's tied to that machine [oxygen].

Recreation and pastimes

As with social life, former recreational pursuits, hobbies and pastimes may be curtailed or abandoned as the illness progresses. As Petty and Nett state: 'Time for recreation . . . is often abundantly available for patients with emphysema'(1984: 101). Hence, in addition to various sedentary activities such as reading, watching television and visiting friends, they also suggest that other, more active pastimes such as gardening, walking, golf, bowling, fishing and swimming may be pursued. Yet, as they themselves also note:

we have observed that many recreational opportunities are not pursued for a variety of reasons. . . . Major reasons are the problems of anxiety, depression, and somatic preoccupation, which permeates the minds and affects the lives and happiness of patients and their families. . . . The same determinants of adjustment that lead to premature abandonment of work are the basic reasons for eliminating or avoiding recreation.

(1984: 101–3)

Indeed, as with social life in general, a number of studies have shown recreation and pastimes to be considerably compromised as a consequence of COAD. For example, as mentioned in Chapter four, McSweeny *et al.* (1982), using the Sickness Impact Profile (SIP), found a reduction of 40 to 50 per cent within this area, whilst the results of Williams' (1990) study suggest a broadly similar picture (see Table 4.1). Moreover, as McSweeny and Labuhn note:

That there is a significant loss of pleasurable activities in [COAD] is relevant to theories of depression which suggest that the loss of reinforcers is a major contributing factor in the development of depression. . . . Therefore, it is possible that helping [COAD] patients to maintain old hobbies or develop new ones might ameliorate the negative impact of the disease on emotional status.

(1990: 402)

Thus Mr Thompson, for example, had, in the past, pursued a variety of recreational activities ranging from cricket, sailing, badminton and golf, through to gardening. Yet, bar the latter, of which he did very little nowadays, he claimed that he had had to give them all up over the years as a consequence of his illness. As he stated:

Well, in the past I mean, I used to play cricket, golf, I had to give that up, the occasional game of badminton, I had to give that up. I mean I used to do quite a lot of sport until my emphysema got worse, you know. I mean, I'd love to be able to play a round of golf still, it's a lovely sort of general exercise golf. I used to play quite a bit of golf, but I couldn't do it now. I mean, if it wasn't for this I certainly would still be playing golf, I said that the other day didn't I [to wife], 'cause a lot of my old cronies still play and I'd still be playing with them, I miss that a great deal. Also I used to do a bit of sailing, I belonged to a sailing club, which was very nice, you know, socially and in every other sense, and I mean we used to go walking didn't we [to wife], you know, we enjoyed going on country walks, but at the end of the day, what can you do?

Yet, as mentioned earlier, the picture is not, or need not be, wholly negative in nature. Rather, whilst certain hobbies, recreational activities and pastimes may be curtailed or forsaken in the wake of chronic illness and disability, it is none the less the case that various other alternative pursuits may be found or suitable substitutes constructed; this being influenced by a variety of other factors in addition to the illness, such as social and material resources, together with the personality, interests, motivation and ingenuity of the individual concerned.

For example, McSweeny *et al.* (1982) found strong correlations between their quality of life measures and COAD patients' age, socio-economic status, neuro-psychological status and exercise tolerance. Similarly, it was also notable how middle-class respondents in Williams' (1990) study tended to fare better than their working-class counterparts in a variety of areas, including the ability to maintain or construct suitable alternative recreation and pastimes. For example, Mrs Prout, a middle-class woman, had taken up antique restoration classes and also managed to keep herself fairly well occupied through reading, letter-writing, card-making (using pressed flowers) and playing the piano. She was also closely involved in her local church from which, she claimed, she derived a good deal of spiritual comfort and inspiration in coping with her illness. Indeed, as Stollenwerk (1985) suggests, patients' spiritual resources should also be assessed for their potential as a coping resource. In her study of self-care practices amongst COAD patients, she found that patients' values and spiritual beliefs affected not only their decisions regarding self-care practices, but also their attitudes and emotional stability. Hence Stollenwerk encourages professionals to become better aware of patients' values in order to assist individuals to achieve their goals.

Holidays

Holidays may also prove to be problematic in the wake of COAD. Indeed, holidays were a common area where problems arose in Williams' (1990) study: 72 per cent stating that COAD had or did cause problems and difficulties regarding their holidays. Similarly, many of those in Nocon and Booth's (1991) study of the social impact of asthma stated that their asthma affected their holiday arrangements.

A wide range of problems and difficulties were mentioned by those in Williams' (1990) study. First, there were the obvious difficulties of attempting to plan and arrange a holiday in the face of a chronic, fluctuating and uncertain illness condition. This, as Mr Thompson pointed out, included the problem of getting holiday insurance. Additional issues included some or all of the following: the problems (both objective and subjective) of travelling; limited indoor and outdoor mobility; the necessity of having to consider the geography, terrain and climatic conditions of the location; the problem of medical regimens, particularly for those on long-term oxygen therapy; and, finally, the sheer amount of time and effort which planning and going on holiday actually involved. Mrs McLeod, for example, nicely summarised some of the problems and difficulties involved in a holiday:

> Wherever you want to go and whatever you want to do you've got a restriction, and I mean, you've got to arrange and plan everything. For instance, you've got to arrange your oxygen, how you're going to get there, whether there's a lift in the hotel, what facilities they've got, what the local environment's like, you know, all sorts of things have to be taken into account, planned for and arranged. You can't do anything on the spur of the moment, I mean it's not like you just put your suitcase in the back of the car and go off somewhere, you know.

Mr Brown, meanwhile, spoke of his fear of flying nowadays:

> Well, I would like to be able to spend the winter months abroad in Spain but, frankly, to be quite honest with you, I'm scared to fly in my condition. 'Cause I mean, if you're on a plane and you have a bad attack . . . I mean, it's bad enough having an attack in your own home, imagine what it would be like when you're 35,000 feet up in the air!

Accounts such as these serve to highlight and reinforce the myriad dimensions of disadvantage COAD sufferers experience as a consequence of the disease and its sequelae. As Mr O'Riley remarked, a holiday would be something to look both forward to and back upon, but, perhaps more importantly, would also help to break up the sheer monotony of his daily existence. Mrs Bush, meanwhile, who was close to breaking point already regarding her husband's illness, exclaimed: 'Oh, to have a holiday would be marvellous. Just to get away from it all, even if it was only for a few days, you know. Please God, I'm hoping we can have one next year.' However, as she conceded, the chance was slim, yet the hope was still important.

Social withdrawal, isolation and confinement

It can be readily appreciated how persistent symptoms of coughing and sputum production, in addition to breathlessness, may cause considerable spoilage of interaction and lead to social withdrawal. As Strauss and others have suggested, withdrawal from social interaction and social life more generally is 'entirely understandable ... given the accompanying symptoms, crises, regimens, and often difficult phasing of trajectories' (1975: 54). Furthermore, as discussed in Chapter two, anxiety-provoking situations tend to trigger breathlessness which then triggers further anxiety, placing the sufferer in a vicious circle which can prove difficult to break out of. Consequently, research has indicated a tendency for COAD patients – both as a response to their symptoms and as an attempt to control or minimise them – to become withdrawn, to avoid social interaction and to rely heavily on the psychological coping mechanism of 'isolation of affect, denial and repression' (Dudley *et al.* 1980).

For example, as has already been noted, Dudley *et al.* (1973) observed that many severely disabled COAD patients tend to live in what they termed 'emotional strait jackets' due to any significant emotional changes triggering distressing symptoms. Similarly, Lester (1973) found that COAD patients tend to opt for what he referred to as a 'constricted living space', both spatially and socially, involving a withdrawal into the home and avoidance of interaction with others. However, such strategies, whilst understandable responses to what are often highly distressing symptoms, are not without their own costs and problems – not the least of which concerns the further restriction of what are already often highly compromised life styles. Indeed, such strategies are often taken as indicators of 'maladjustment' *vis-à-vis* 'adjustment' to COAD.

Such strategies also proved, in varying degrees, to be a common response, or 'mode of adaptation', for COAD sufferers in Williams' (1990) study. Whilst 21 per cent stated that they never or only rarely found themselves avoiding social situations or interactions with others due to their breathing problems (as distinct from reasons of embarrassment), 59 per cent admitted to sometimes doing this and a further 21 per cent stated that they often found themselves doing so. Thus sufferers frequently spoke of having to avoid any sort of 'anxiety-provoking' or 'stressful situations', of trying to avoid emotionally charged situations, and of limiting the amount of company they had and the amount of socialising they did. Mr King, for example, admitted to avoiding situations which were likely to lead to him getting 'tensed-up', 'excited' or 'nervous' and hence more breathless:

> almost any sort of a situation where there's any kind of excitement or whatever, I can't get involved in it. Because if I have to breathe

anything above what I know is required to keep me in some kind of a stable condition, if I get anything above that, I become paralysed, it's as simple as that. . . . So you've got to avoid situations involving any kind of excitement or anything like that.

Mr Tucker, meanwhile, provided a particularly good example of a 'maladaptive' response. He appeared to be highly anxious, frightened and distressed regarding his illness – particularly the breathlessness and the threat of sudden attacks. Consequently, he did indeed appear to live most of his life in a social and emotional 'strait jacket', largely confining himself to the house, where he claimed to feel safer, having all his medication ready to hand in the event of an 'emergency'.

Others spoke of the sheer physical and mental effort involved in attempting to maintain any sort of social life and in trying to be sociable – particularly if they still worked and had to invest their limited energy reserves in trying to hold down a job. As Mr Brown stated:

I don't want too much of people nowadays. Now my wife, she loves talking to people but, these days, as a consequence of my illness I suppose, 'cause I never used to be like it, I find that after a while I've had enough of people. I don't mind passing the time of day, but I don't want to spend any length of time with them. . . . No I don't like company for any length of time, I find I can't take it nowadays . . .

An inability to get out and about as much and as easily compared to the past, together with a curtailment of social life, may bring in its wake a *subjective* feeling – whether objectively correct or not – of social isolation and of being cut off from the flux of everyday social life outside the home. Furthermore, as Charmaz found in her study of the chronically ill:

Lack of participation in work alone resulted in social isolation for most of those interviewed. Few had intimate relationships beyond those developed through work and family. Earlier friendships usually waned as ill persons no longer shared the same social worlds.

(1983: 176)

COAD sufferers in Williams' (1990) study were asked whether, and if so how often, they experienced *feelings* of loneliness and social isolation. Whilst 36 per cent said that they 'never' or only 'rarely' had such feelings, 45 per cent admitted to 'sometimes' feeling this way and a further 20 per cent said that they 'often' felt this. For example, Mr Charlton claimed that he had not been out for the last six weeks and that he was 'just about getting fed up with it'. This situation was further exacerbated by the necessity of his wife having to work full-time. Consequently, he was left in the flat on his own all day long with little or nothing to occupy his time and fill his days. As he tellingly put it when asked whether he felt socially isolated and cut off from the world outside:

Sometimes, yeah sometimes I do. I sit here don't I [to wife] and I look at these four walls and I just wanna get out, you know, when I've been stuck indoors for a time and I ain't seen nobody much, then I do don't I [to wife], particularly when she's at work all day long. Like now really, 'cause I ain't been out of the house for six weeks now have I [to wife]? It's like being in prison 'in it, it's like you're doing time for a crime you didn't commit, well not wittingly at least. But at least in prison you have got someone to talk to, you understand what I mean, but here I've got no one to talk to 'cause if no one's here, no one's here are they? You feel sort of cut off, everybody who's in the same boat as me gets that feeling, I mean they must do, I don't care who they are, I know I do, I get that feeling don't I [to wife]?

In such contexts, days may prove difficult to fill and a strong sense of monotony, boredom and frustration may sometimes follow. Days merge imperceptibly one into another. Thus Mr O'Riley stated:

Well, it's hard to tell one day from the next really to be honest with you, they're all the same to me now. In fact, if I didn't have a paper and watch the news on the telly I don't think I'd know what day of the week it was tell you the truth . . . they're all the same to me now.

And Mr Doyal remarked:

Well, it's just living, just existing, that's all. . . . You just have to learn to live a new, different, type of life than what I used to, you know, completely re-adjust.

Meanwhile, concerning the issue of monotony in his daily existence, Mr O'Riley again remarked:

Yeah, I feel that it gets monotonous all right, yeah. But there's not a lot, you know, not a lot you can do about it, what can you do like. I try to ah, you know, forget about those feelings, try to get 'em out of me mind and think about something else, 'cause if you're going to keep mulling it over in your mind and worrying about things like that, you're going to make yourself worse, drive yourself crazy aren't you. I make meself worse, I know that, really, I do make meself worse.

When you think of what you was able to do in the past and what you have been doing lately, stuck at home here with nothing to do 'cept watch the television, bored out of your skull, it ah, it makes you feel very depressed, very depressed and miserable sometimes.

This, however, is not to suggest a wholly negative picture. Rather, as Petty and Nett (1984), amongst others, have suggested, despite the severity of the illness, it remains possible that COAD sufferers – particularly those with strong 'psychosocial assets', supportive social networks, and financial and material resources (including access to a car) – may still, in the face of this progressively disabling disease, be able to get out and about, maintain contact with the outside world, engage in various forms of recreation and pastimes, and hence lead, at least in part, a meaningful and fulfilling life. Unfortunately, however, the frightening and progressively disabling nature of COAD's symptomatology, together with the fact that it disproportionately affects those from working-class backgrounds who may be least able to cope with its consequences, all too often tends to militate against such a 'positive adaptation' to the disease process.

STIGMA, TOLERANCE AND LEGITIMACY

Stigma and embarrassment

As writers as diverse as Darwin (1895/1955) and Goffman (1963) have emphasised, the expression of emotions and the potential for embarrassment are fundamental aspects of both human nature and social interaction (Schudson 1984). In this respect, as Elias's (1978) analysis of manners and the civilising process shows, respiratory symptoms are anathema to many of our contemporary codes of conduct, and our sense of what is deemed 'correct' behaviour and 'good' manners. Thus breathlessness, coughing and sputum production tend to violate tacit, yet culturally entrenched, social expectations, codes of etiquette and decorum, found deeply embedded within routine social interaction. Moreover, as discussed below in the section on tolerance and legitimacy, COAD represents one of a range of chronic conditions which has little appeal to public sentiments. This presents additional problems and a further twist to the already spiralling social disadvantage which sufferers commonly experience as a consequence of the disease.

Thus Guyatt et al. (1987), for example, found embarrassment regarding symptoms, disability and medication to be important dimensions of experience for many of the COAD patients within their study. Similarly, the vast majority of those in Williams' (1990) study stated that they suffered embarrassment regarding either their symptoms, their disability, or their medication (e.g. inhalers, nebulisers or oxygen) when in public. However, medication proved to be less embarrassing, particularly amongst older people, whilst women generally tended to feel more embarrassed than men.

Scambler (1989), in his study of epilepsy, draws a key distinction between what he terms 'felt' and 'enacted' stigma: that is to say, the difference between an individual's perceived sense of stigma and actual occurrences of stigmatisation by others. For most of those within Williams' (1990) study, it was the former rather than the latter type of stigma which was most frequently experienced. Thus, concerning the embarrassing nature of symptoms, Mr Brown stated:

'cause bear in mind, what I do here, which I find natural in my own home, if you was to do that when you were outside, people would immediately turn round and look, especially when you're coughing and trying to clear your chest, the sound of it coming up is anathema to other people. . . . You're an embarrassment to people, they are embarrassed and so are you when you're coughing and spluttering, you know, trying to clear your chest. I mean it's not a nice noise to make, even my wife doesn't enjoy hearing me do it and she's used to it, oh it's terrible.

Meanwhile, concerning disability and mobility-related problems when in public – sometimes resulting in various forms of 'enacted' stigma – Mrs McLeod remarked:

Well, I used to get a bit embarrassed when I was more mobile and I had to keep stopping for breath, as people used to stare. 'Cause I mean, you'd have to stop for breath, you know, and people would look at you as if to say, well once I was taken for a drunk. I was walking along the road to me mum's and I had to stop for breath, and so I leaned up against the wall and I had me head down, and someone come along and said 'That's what you get for standing in the pubs all day.' Oh it was awful, I felt so embarrassed, but at the same time quite angry, you know. I mean, I could have been really ill but no one come up and asked if I was OK. But when I finally did get to me mum's and I thought about it, I could see how they could think I was drunk, it had never occurred to me before, but you can see how people could think that can't you?

A more subtle problem, raised by Mrs Thompson below, concerned the sense of embarrassment and shame male sufferers felt when their wives had to struggle carrying heavy bags of shopping or luggage whilst, to the casual observer, they appeared to be uncaringly strolling along unencumbered:

Mrs Thompson: But you [Mr Thompson] don't like it do you when, like last week, we had a couple of days away. Well Ken [Mr Thompson] can't carry the cases any more and so I had to carry them, and you don't like that do you?

Mr Thompson: No, I don't like things like that, it's embarrassing isn't it, I get very self-conscious and upset about that.

As mentioned earlier, medical regimens may also prove to be a source of considerable embarrassment. Many of those in Williams' (1990) study spoke of how they preferred to use their inhalers discreetly when out of public view, retiring to the toilet or some other clandestine place so as to avoid a potentially 'embarrassing incident' (Goffman 1963). Some also spoke of how they felt others perceived them as 'junkies' or 'drug addicts' when forced to use their medication in full public view. However, one of the main sources of embarrassment regarding medical regimens proved to be the use of things such as nebulisers and oxygen therapy. Thus, concerning oxygen therapy, Mrs White stated:

Well I do get a bit embarrassed to be quite honest with you, particularly with strangers, or people that don't know me. For instance, with some of my husband's friends say, who have had no prior warning of what to expect like, I have to arrange to let them know about it first. 'Cause otherwise I think to meself: 'Well what are they gonna think with me walkin' in with a blimmin' great oxygen cylinder and what have you', you know. So I have to arrange to let them know beforehand, given them prior warning of what to expect like. And I mean, when I'm out in public, if ever I go shopping, especially children, they tend to stare at the portable oxygen cylinder and that 'strange' pipe which disappears up my nose, and often their mothers'll sort of pull them away from you, you know.

Well, I was in a lift in a store with my mum a while ago, and a woman got in with a small child and he kept asking 'What's that up that lady's nose mum?' and you could see she was getting embarrassed. Anyway, in the end she took him out of the lift, she wouldn't let him come in the lift with me. Rather than try to explain, she chose to walk up the stairs with him instead. I've had people walk around rather than past me, perhaps they think I've got AIDS or something, something catching! But other people just look at you and smile.

Faced with such problems and difficulties, strategies may have to be devised in an attempt to deal with or overcome them. Thus, regarding mobility-related problems in public, for example, one of the most frequently mentioned strategies by those in Williams' (1990) study was to 'window shop' and 'look inconspicuous' so as to avoid drawing attention to oneself whenever the necessity to stop for breath arose. As Mr Thompson put it:

Yes you do, yes you do [get embarrassed], ah, you tend to 'window shop' quite a lot, you know, you tend to look in the shop window which contains not the slightest thing of interest to you at all – well, I've never been a great shopper at the best of times anyway, so the last thing I want to do is look in shops! But I do find if I'm out that I tend to do a lot of 'window shopping' which, decoded, is really getting your breath back without being too obvious to all and sundry who happen to be around at the time, you know.

Another strategy which some adopted was to walk at a distance in front, behind or on the other side of the road from whoever they were with: first, in order to avoid drawing attention to their slowness of pace compared to a 'normal lunger' (Fagerhaugh 1975); and, second, so as to avoid the embarrassment of others seeing them empty handed whilst their companions, particularly wives, were weighed down with heavy bags or luggage. As mentioned above, other strategies included the strategic management of information regarding both the illness and medical regimens. Yet all such strategies lead, via their varied and tortuous routes, in one and the same direction: namely, the general desire to appear 'normal'. As Mr Bush put it:

I'm very self-conscious I suppose about me illness, I get very embarrassed about it. I like people to think I'm 'normal', not an invalid. I just want to appear as 'normal' as possible.

Issues of tolerance and legitimacy

It is in contexts such as those described above that issues of legitimacy, tolerance and the understanding of others towards the chronically sick and disabled loom large. As Locker states in his study of rheumatoid arthritis sufferers:

One problem common to many of the respondents, and there are some who would argue that it is common to all who lay claim to an acute or chronic illness . . . is that of legitimation – having others accept the reality of their distress and the inevitability of the constraints imposed upon them. This requires others to define their complaints as valid indicators of subjective experiences and their incapacity as disability created by a chronic condition and not wilful deviance. . . . The problem is not, as Parsons' original discussion might suggest, confined to the prediagnostic stage of the disease; it is never wholly resolved by the provision of a clinical label. . . . Doctors and other accredited gatekeepers may separate the disabled from the deviant during the diagnostic process but family, friends, colleagues and strangers, even co-sufferers, while accepting the person's status as disabled, continue to monitor his or her performance in that role. The meaning of the diagnosis fluctuates, being negotiated and renegotiated over time.

(1983: 131)

Similarly, Charmaz notes that:

Others generally view the chronically ill through the framework of acute care with its assumptions of illness causing temporary disruptions of self rather than causing continued losses of self. Hence, others' realization of their suffering tends to be absent, limited or minimized.

(1983: 169)

Nowhere is this more so than in relation to COAD.

As Bury notes, the experience of chronic illness involves 'testing structures of support and risking meanings within the practical constraints of home and work' (1988: 92). Whilst, on the one hand, the largely 'invisible', intangible, nature of the COAD may be a positive asset, enabling sufferers to 'pass as normal', on the other hand, it may also create considerable problems. COAD represents one of a range of chronic conditions which has little appeal to public sentiments, in contrast to areas such as the health of sick children or cancer. The stereotypical image of a breathless, wheezing, coughing, spitting and spluttering (old) man suffering a chronic respiratory disease – which is firmly linked in the public mind with smoking – is greeted with relatively little public sympathy compared to that of, say, a sick child struck down by a malevolent disease, or a young adult confined to a wheelchair. Moreover, even when 'responsibility' for causing the disease (e.g. smoking) is laid aside, the issue of culpability may still be projected forward onto how the individual actually copes with the disease (Williams and Bury 1989a).

In Williams' (1990) study, for example, issues of legitimacy, tolerance and the understanding of others towards COAD were major themes in sufferers' accounts. Many spoke of how they felt the legitimacy of their condition was either overtly or covertly challenged by others, and of the lack of understanding of others regarding the reality of their predicament. As Mr Thompson appositely remarked: 'The first thing you have to remember when talking about people with respiratory illness, is that you have to cut off one of their legs before anybody realises they are disabled!' He continued:

Well I think most people, when they understand the problem, are very considerate. But of course, you know, if you see a 'healthy' looking fellow strolling across the road, you expect them to be 'healthy', you know, and you expect them to be able to give you a hand on the bus if you're an old lady and these sorts of things. But with this thing you just can't do it and it does cause a lot of misunderstanding and embarrassment because, to the casual observer, you look, to all intents and purposes, quite normal, fit and healthy.

I mean, I was standing in a queue in a DIY shop and the chap in front of me was disabled. The shop was busy and this chap wanted a bag of charcoal. So he asked the shop assistant if he would mind carrying it out to his car for him. Well, as I say, the shop was busy. . . . So he [shop assistant] suggested that perhaps the chap behind, which happened to be me, might kindly carry it to the car instead. Well of course, this put me in a very difficult and embarrassing position, because I then had to explain that unfortunately I couldn't as my health was not very good either . . . it was all very embarrassing as I felt and got the distinct impression that nobody really understood or believed me and that consequently they thought I was just being bloody minded and selfish, you know, that I just couldn't be bothered to help this poor chap.

Mr Bush remarked:

Well sittin' here now I appear the picture of health don't I? You see, unless you're on crutches, in a wheelchair or swathed in bandages, people don't seem to understand. Actually I've been called a 'fraud' before now, you know, yeah [laughs], half joking like, but all the same, I've had it said: 'You're a "fraud", look at you there's nothing the matter with you', oh yeah. Tell 'em you've got cancer or that you've had a heart attack or something like that and they're very sympathetic and understanding, but tell 'em you've got emphysema and they look

at you blank like. . . . Or they'll say: 'Oh yes, I've had a bit of
bronchitis or chest trouble myself, I suffer with a weak chest', you
know, that sort of thing. They just don't seem to understand the extent
of it.

Mr Brown, meanwhile, spoke at length of how he found the legitimacy
of his condition a problem:

Well, for instance, I'm thinking of getting a mobile scooter thing, you
know, for disabled people, I was going to get one this year. But that's
all very well for people who have got obvious signs of disability, but
when I'm sitting down, I appear to be quite 'normal' and 'healthy'. So
if, say, I had a scooter and I got where I wanted to go and I got off and
walked away, people would say: 'Well what's he got that for, he
doesn't need that'. . . . And so I feel that if I got a scooter people would
think I was a fraud, and that if people asked me, I'd have to explain
that it's all very well whilst I'm sitting down or doing nothing active – I
appear to be as 'normal' as the next person then – but that they should
see me after I've crossed the road, or done anything active. You've got
to explain your illness or your disability away all the time . . .

Now if you turned round and you told 'em you had something
terminal like cancer, or that you were suffering from something which
was recognised as being very disabling like multiple sclerosis, oh well
then they'd all be very sympathetic. But tell 'em you've got chest
trouble or severe bronchitis and it's a very different story, they don't
seem to understand. I suppose it's because they think it's an ordinary
everyday illness that most people have got anyway, or at least have
suffered from in some degree, shape or form. I mean, there are times
when even normal, healthy people over-exert themselves and get a bit
breathless, so others may, on seeing you like that, just think to
themselves you've just done exactly the same thing, when in point of
fact, you're in the middle of a bad attack. But if you do attempt to tell
other people, try to explain what's the matter with you, very often all
you get is something like: 'Oh I'm a bit chesty myself', or; 'Oh my
little grandson Johnny sufferers with asthma', you know. They just
don't seem to understand what you're up against.

Similarly, note the following remarks by Mrs Charlton regarding her
husband's condition and the tolerance and understanding of her
workmates:

Mrs Charlton: . . . like in work like, the women know my husband's ill
and they see him up at the window – 'cause I only work

over there [factory over the road] – and they said: 'He looks all right to me', Pat and Hilda. And so I said: 'But he's not.' But they said: 'He looks well to me, I see him up at the window, he looks well!'

Mr Charlton: Yeah, I've had a few people like that.

Mrs Charlton: I mean me, I look like this all the time, white and everything else like that, you know, and they say to me 'You look ill', but when it comes to him, they don't understand – I think they think it's terrible me going to work with him at home like, like he's swinging the lead, you know. They said to me: 'Oh, he don't half look well your husband.' Well I just shook me head in disbelief, you can't seem to get it through to them that he's ill, they think you're kidding or something, that he's trying it on, bone idle or something like that, you know.

Mr Charlton: Yeah, that's what I'm saying, like a lot of people look at you and you can see 'em thinking or they'll say: 'Cor, you don't half look well, there's nothing wrong with you.' And you think to yourself, I don't wanna start losing me temper 'cause that's when I start getting breathless. So I just walk away quietly muttering something, you know, 'cause there's little point in trying to explain to people like that. I just walk away.

Of course, as we shall see in the section on family life below, such 'limits of tolerance' and understanding are not merely restricted to the wider public realm, they may also extend into the domestic and family milieux.

SOCIAL SUPPORT AND SOCIAL CONTACT

As Locker (1983) notes, whilst the main source of help and support concerning chronic illness and disability tends to come from the family, particularly spouses and daughters (Blaxter 1976, Moroney 1976), it is none the less the case that helper and helped exist within wider social networks which may be more or less supportive. Indeed, the presence or absence of wider social support networks may have an important influence upon how sufferers and their families adapt to and manage their condition. Jensen (1983), for instance, in a study of the role of social support and various risk factors in COAD patients' symptom management, found that social support and life stress were better predictors of the number of hospitalisations than the patient's demographic characteristics, illness severity or previous hospitalisations.

In Young's (1982) study, however, the availability of such support was not found to be directly related to COAD patients' self-adaptation, but it was found to have a significant effect upon the spouses' adaptation. However, only 20 per cent of patients reported that they received assistance from persons other than their spouses and immediate family, which may account for the greater importance of such support for the spouses in Young's study. Indeed, approximately two-thirds of spouses in Sexton and Monro's (1985) study said that they relied heavily upon their sons and daughters for help. As McSweeny and Labuhn (1990) note, these findings suggest that most COAD patients 'rely heavily upon their immediate families for support whilst family members may rely on each other as well as professional and community resources' (1990: 404).

Few of those in Williams' (1990) study reported actually having received much in the way of practical help and assistance from their social networks. Indeed, only 27 per cent of those who possessed a social support network were currently receiving help and support of this nature; these tending to be those who, for various reasons, lived on their own, particularly men. The remainder were not in receipt of such help. There are of course many reasons why wider social support networks are not mobilised or drawn upon, ranging from pride, a desire for independence, and not wanting to over-burden already busy family lives, through to an ability to cope adequately without outside help and support. However, as others have suggested (Finch and Groves 1983, Anderson 1988), the main responsibility and burden of care seems to rest with the spouse and immediate family, and although this is often given willingly, it can be both emotionally and physically demanding. As Barstow (1974) found in her study, COAD patients identified the presence of a supportive spouse as the most important factor in successful coping, whilst Sexton and Monro (1988) reported similar findings in their study of female sufferers.

Many studies have also documented the decline and loss of social contact, the withering of wider social support networks, and the subsequent sense of isolation which chronic illness and disability may bring in its wake. In this respect disadvantage is not simply a matter of material deprivation, but also involves the degree to which the chronically sick and disabled are able to maintain contact with the outside world and their links with wider social networks. In Williams' (1990) study, for example, many sufferers, even those who possessed a wider social network, spoke of how their networks and overall degree of social contact had considerably diminished since their illness first began. This was particularly the case concerning so-called 'friends' as opposed to kin. Thus Miss Bell, for example, who lived alone, remarked:

> Well, I had lots of friends at one time, but I've found that gradually, since I've been ill and I've stopped work, they've stayed away, you know, they don't visit so much, they've gradually dwindled away. I mean, I've slowly found out who my *real* true friends are since I've been ill, you know, and that's been very upsetting, a very upsetting experience indeed. You know, gradually I've lost touch, gradually they'd start making excuses as to why they hadn't been in touch. I'd even see them going past my flat and not popping in and I couldn't believe it at first. I thought: 'How could they do it to me? Why is it?' And when I asked them they just made up excuses or said: 'Oh well, it's just one of those things', you know. But I mean, I think it's because you can't do the things you used to be able to do, you're a liability to others when you're ill aren't you, and they're frightened to get involved; too busy with their own lives for illness.

Mr Thomas, meanwhile, whose wife was also chronically ill and disabled, stated:

> Well we ain't got no one really, no one really, not now. Since we've both become ill they've [friends] all gone up in a puff of smoke, they just seem to have fizzled out. Friends just seem to drop off for some reason when you're ill, they don't seem to wanna know.

Other potential sources of social contact and social support, of course, concern the church, together with various voluntary bodies, organisations and self-help groups (Morgan *et al.* 1985). As McSweeny and Labuhn state:

> Many patients and relatives will also find peer support groups to be very helpful. In the United States these include the Better Breathers Clubs, which are supported by the local chapters of the American Lung Association. These groups usually include discussions of psychosocial issues as well as educational programs concerning medical aspects of [COAD]. Practical information such as the location of restaurants with no-smoking policies is often available through these groups.
>
> (1990: 413)

Yet, to the authors' knowledge, no such extensive, well established and well organised network of self-help groups specifically for COAD sufferers and their families exists in the United Kingdom to date. One possible exception is the 'Breathe Easy' club run by the British Lung Foundation. The British Lung Foundation was launched in 1985 by a group of chest physicians in order to raise funds for research into lung disease, and also to increase public awareness of the extent of lung disease and the importance of 'good' respiratory health. 'Breathe Easy' is a club for those with long-term breathing problems. Members of this club receive a regular newsletter providing up-to-date information on lung conditions, treatments and services available, and so on. A further aim is to encourage and facilitate the sharing of information and experiences amongst people in similar situations.

As Morgan *et al.* (1985) note, the general question of why self-help groups are more prevalent in the United States than in Western Europe has been explained in terms of differences in attitude and value between the two societies – the United States placing greater emphasis upon individual responsibility for development and destiny, together with differences in health and welfare provision. However, regarding COAD in particular, it may also be the case that self-help activities are fairly limited due to: the nature of the condition as such; the tendency for patients to become socially withdrawn and limit social interaction as the disease progresses; the reluctance of many COAD sufferers to see themselves as 'disabled'; problems of stigma, legitimacy and tolerance of others towards the condition; and, finally, COAD's association with deprived occupational and social circumstances. Indeed, the general picture which emerged in Williams' (1990) UK study was of COAD sufferers and their families having fairly limited contact with, and involvement in, any such organisations or self-help groups, other than the church, which may have existed. Such a situation served to isolate them still further, both from the wider society and from fellow sufferers.

MARRIAGE AND FAMILY LIFE

As has been emphasised throughout the course of this book, chronic illness and disability are not isolated phenomena whose consequences are merely restricted to the sufferer. Rather, as Locker notes:

> It is now common for helping professionals or others who have dealings with chronically sick people to talk of the 'disabled family' in recognition that the effects of a long-term illness extend beyond the individual afflicted to envelop their close associates. . . . While disability disables the normal by rendering rules of social interaction inapplicable, it also has longer term effects on others, particularly

family members, whose daily lives may be severely dislocated by the presence of a disabled person in the household.

(1983: 155)

As Bruhn (1977) suggests, chronic illness is more likely to be disintegrative rather than integrative for families. As duties, roles and responsibilities are gradually taken over by others, the chronically ill may experience a profound sense of loss, whilst other family members may feel over-burdened. Similarly, in reviewing the literature on COAD, McSweeny and Labuhn (1990) conclude that, like most other chronic conditions, it tends to have a negative impact upon both sufferers' and their families' quality of life.

Yet, in common with many other forms of chronic illness, much of the day-to-day reality and experience of coping with COAD goes on 'behind closed doors' in a context of considerable stress and strain, uncertainty and anxiety. As Bury notes:

Relationships do not guarantee particular responses, indeed it is the response that shapes the relationships. . . . Individuals and their families cannot be entirely sure what the event of such an illness means or will mean for the future; meanings are fashioned in the flux of change, as events unfold.

(1988: 92)

Thus, as Bury concludes:

Working in a situation of considerable uncertainty . . . individuals, families and others frequently test the limits of the strength of their relationships, particularly the amount of support and care they are able or willing to afford each other.

(1988: 113)

Moreover, COAD sufferers and their families often have very different perceptions of both the nature of the problems posed by the illness and the sufferers' capabilities. For example, Guyatt *et al.* (1987) had thirty-six pairs of sufferers and their significant others complete an identical questionnaire about problems posed by the illness covering areas such as dyspnoea, mastery, fatigue, sleep disturbance, emotional problems, social problems and cognitive function. Whilst patients identified more of the items as problematic than the significant others, the latter attached greater importance to the problems which they identified and the correlation between patient and relative total scores were only moderate. As McSweeny and Labuhn (1990) note, these differing views, attitudes and expectations of patients and family members may also contribute to sufferers' feelings of isolation, depression and their ability to cope, as well as to carers' own subjective feelings of (di)stress. This underlines the importance of physicians taking into account patient and family views of illness-related problems rather than relying solely upon physical indicators of disease (McSweeny and Labuhn 1990).

If a general picture of marriage and family life emerged in Williams (1990) study, it was of marriages having survived the test of time in the wake of COAD. This may, of course, be partly artefactual, due to the tendency for COAD to occur in middle to later life, by which time the majority of marriages still in existence would, presumably, be fairly solid and robust. Indeed, the vast majority of those who were married spoke of and rated their spouses as having been very helpful and supportive to them since the onset of their illness condition – although the response was generally less enthusiastic, though still positive, concerning other family members. Spouses, both male and female, were often singled out for praise with comments such as the following: 'Well, I mean, she's been everything, she's been me right arm . . . I couldn't manage without her'; 'Oh, she's been marvellous, very good'; and 'Oh he's been very good, oh yes, very tolerant, very helpful and supportive.' Thus, Mrs Prout remarked of her daughter and husband:

> And my daughter, she's my friend, she's always been very supportive, very kind and very, very understanding and that's true of my husband also. I don't know what I would do without him, I'm not just talking about all the help he does around the house, I also mean as a friend. I don't know how I would get on without him because he understands me totally, you know, we are totally one.

Similarly, patients in Barstow's (1974) study identified the presence of a supportive spouse as the most important factor in successful coping; 40 per cent of Hanson's (1982) patients claimed that COAD had had a positive impact on their marriage; whilst 95 per cent of female sufferers in Sexton and Monro's (1988) study identified their husbands as important sources of support. In particular, husbands provided instrumental support by helping out with various household tasks and activities, treatments and other things required. In addition, approximately half of these women claimed that they talked their problems over with their husbands, and also turned to friends, relatives and children for emotional support. Interestingly, however, despite the support given by husbands and families, approximately one-third still said that they felt lonely and depressed. Also, in another interesting study,

Labuhn (1984) found that married COAD patients had better exercise tolerance than single, widowed or divorced patients even after controlling for age, disease severity and neuro-psychological functioning. Although marriage did not have a significant impact upon patients' depressed mood states, it indirectly contributed to patients' physical and psychosocial functioning through its impact on their exercise capacity.

One of the main sources of tension and difficulty regarding family life identified by those in Williams' (1990) study arose from the sheer sense of frustration and irritability the illness tended to create which, at times, was vented on those closest to hand (i.e. their 'nearest and dearest'). As Goffman notes in relation to mental illness within the family: 'The home, where wounds are meant to be licked, becomes precisely the place where they are inflicted. Boundaries are broken. The family is turned inside out' (1971: 381). Thus Mrs Prout, again, remarked:

> Unfortunately, I do, sometimes, not all the time, but sometimes, I go off my head and I say things that haven't even any truth in them about my family. And it's sheer, some people would say it's temper, but it's sheer frustration, because I can't do the things I normally do. Maybe I've had a frustrating day where I've wanted to do a lot of things and I couldn't do them, or maybe somebody's said something that's triggered me off, and it's just like a firework going off, and I'm so sorry afterwards. And then I'll go for a time and I'm very placid, I am quite placid you know. And, ah, we have such a good relationship, the family, that I don't want to spoil it and there I go, you know, off my head, and it's frustration, sheer frustration, that's all.

Mr Charlton also confessed to being short tempered:

Mr Charlton: ... and it [the illness], it gets you so frustrated and irritable at times that you're inclined to lose your temper and take it out on your nearest and dearest. Oh yeah, terrible.

Mrs Charlton: Yeah, you're treading on eggshells with him sometimes when he gets like that, you know.

Mr Charlton: Yeah, I'm swearing and cursing and God knows what to be honest. I'm not proud of it, but it gets you that way sometimes.

Similarly, the major problem for the wives of COAD sufferers in Sexton and Monro's (1985) study was of being worried about their husbands' condition, his negative attitudes and irritability, and coping with the loss of their own freedom. Less than one-third said that they shared their problems with their husbands as most were afraid that this would lead to their husbands having an attack of dyspnoea.

As Shearer (1981) notes, the relationship between helper and helped is one fraught with difficulties, many of which are not easily resolved. In such contexts, helper and helped are placed in a situation of considerable uncertainty, ambiguity and tension. Willingly offered help can be curtly rejected as a symbol of 'dependency' or 'incompetence', whilst no such offers may equally be construed as 'uncaring'. Thus a 'double bind', or a situation of 'mutual handicap', results in which the disabled may feel unable to ask for help, whilst others may also feel unable to offer it in ways which do not create tensions and difficulties for both.

As mentioned earlier, the main responsibility and burden of care tends to rest with the immediate family, predominantly the spouse. Yet as Anderson (1988) has recently suggested in relation to those caring for stroke victims, such caring can develop into an 'unremitting burden'. In Rubeck's (1971) study of fifty male bronchitics, for example, wives often reported symptoms such as exhaustion, insomnia, recurrent migraine and 'nerves'. Similarly, wives of COAD sufferers in Sexton and Monro's (1985) study reported many difficulties with sleeping due to their husbands' breathing problems. They had also taken on many extra responsibilities and given up many of their own social activities as a consequence of their husbands' illness.

There were also a number of examples in Williams' (1990) study of how the stresses and strains of the caring role had taken their toll physically, psychologically and socially. Mrs Bush, for example, appeared to be both physically and mentally exhausted as a consequence of her caring role, and suffered with 'headaches and psoriasis'; both of which she claimed were brought on by 'me nerves'. As she put it:

> I can't even be out for very long, I can't leave him on his own for more than three-quarters of an hour at the most and then only if he says that he's feeling OK. . . . He's totally dependent on me now, and I mean, he wouldn't go and stay with me daughter to give me a bit of a break, he's odd like that.

Similarly, Mrs Tucker claimed to be exhausted both mentally and physically by her caring role. Yet it was the restrictions which it placed upon both their lives, coupled with the tensions, difficulties and dilemmas the illness created within the home environment, which she found the hardest to bear and live with:

> Well, there's no let up, there just seems to be no end to it all really, you

know, he's very dependent on me these days. And I mean, I don't wish to sound selfish, but I'm as much trapped indoors as he is these days because, I mean, he doesn't like me going out and leaving him in here alone, you know – well, neither do I for that matter 'cause I tend to worry and I have to hurry back. . . . You know, there just seems to be no light at the end of the tunnel. And I do feel I need a break at times, 'cause it's very wearing. That sounds terrible I know, but it does, it gets very wearing at times, you know. . . . And I mean, you have to be so careful what you say to him at times, you know, 'cause he's inclined to be a bit 'short tempered' these days on account of the illness. I mean I know he can't help it, but when he gets like that, well, you're creeping round the house, watchin' what you say, tryin' not to upset him, you know. It's sheer frustration I know, but it's very difficult to live with at times all the same.

It is in such contexts that, as Charmaz (1983) has highlighted, along with the leading of restricted lives, discreditation and feelings of social isolation, one of the major potential sources of suffering which the chronically ill experience is that of dependency and of feeling a burden upon others. Indeed, feelings of dependency and of being a burden were quite commonly experienced amongst both male and female COAD sufferers in Williams' (1990) study: whilst 27 per cent stated that they 'never' felt a burden to others around them, 46 per cent admitted to 'sometimes' feeling this way, and a further 26 per cent confessed to 'often' feeling a burden. As Mrs Prout remarked:

It has been difficult for me to accept, because I've always been a fairly independent sort of person and I like to do things for people, so I do feel very dependent on them now, a burden to them, and I do worry about that. I mean I just see them working so hard and, ah, doing so much for me. . . . And I feel that my demands, no I don't demand, but I feel as if I am demanding, that my demands are too great on the family unit.

Mrs White, meanwhile, stated:

I feel a lot of the time that I'm holding him back, you know. My husband never really complains, but I'm sure it's a put up thing, that he's putting on a brave face for my benefit sort of thing . . . I mean, he can't go out of the house with me without having to lug oxygen cylinders about. . . . When he's out he's got to make sure I'm all right, leave a phone number in case I want him. . . . The fact that he can't get out when he wants to and as much as he wants to, and get away for a holiday and things like that, you know. He's restricted too you see, but he never really complains, although I know damned well it must get him down at times, it must get on his nerves . . . I think I worry about his freedom more than mine, 'cause I know I'm restricted but he's not.

There were also various examples in Williams' (1990) study of how challenges, sometimes implicit, sometimes explicit, were made by family members regarding not only the legitimacy and reality of the condition as such, but also the distress which sufferers experienced. Such examples served to illustrate how family members' 'limits of tolerance' (Bury 1982, 1988) may be (quickly) reached in the face of a chronic, disabling illness such as COAD. Thus Mr Swain, for example, lived in a situation of considerable friction, tension and conflict, caused in no small part through the general intolerance and lack of understanding of his wife and son. Moreover, the situation was made worse by the fact that his son smoked, and generally appeared to have no real regard for his father's chest condition – something which further served to fuel an already highly charged situation. Such factors added to Mr Swain's own crippling sense of frustration and anguish regarding both his illness and his family's response to it, and further undermined his sense of personal potency within the home, together with his self-esteem and sense of selfhood. Similar feelings were expressed by Mrs Cole regarding her husband and children:

Mrs Cole: Well at first it was, ah, you know, at first he [husband] didn't seem to appreciate the way that I felt, you know, it was hard at first. But now, as the condition has progressed and it's got worse, well I think he understands now. At first he didn't seem to understand that I was ill and that I couldn't do all the things I used to do, I don't think he could accept that in the early stages, things were a bit difficult then. But as time's gone on I think he's become more aware and understanding, he's learnt to accept my limitations sort of thing and he's very helpful.

Mr Cole: The children don't realise how ill she is, you know. I do *now*, but the children don't . . .

Mrs Cole: Because you look well. . . . Because you look well and you get about, you know, and you're going up and down the stairs adequately, you know what I mean, they don't think there's much wrong. . . . Yeah see, you've got to sit in a wheelchair before they see that anything is wrong with you, you know. . . . I feel as if I gotta keep like, apologising, because they look at me as if there's nothing wrong with me, you know what I mean. I know I'm not dying or, but nobody can appreciate the way I feel, you know. I tell 'em, but they don't necessarily, they look at you as if you're lying, do you know what I mean, or they just make you feel as if you're putting it on or something or, you know. I mean I'm not looking for sympathy, just a little bit of understanding and tolerance.

Of course, another major dimension of quality of life in general and marriage and family life in particular concerns the issue of sexuality and the quality of the sexual relationship. The problems and difficulties COAD creates regarding sufferers' sex lives, particularly in the latter stages of the disease, may be profound. The decline in sexual drive, capacity and ability consequent upon COAD may cause profound psychosocial problems for sufferers, and such difficulties require a sympathetic and understanding spouse or partner. Thus, as Petty and Nett note, COAD patients' sex lives are affected:

by either real or perceived sexual limitation or by actual failure to function for both men and women in various stages in the development of [COAD]. Many men have difficulty achieving or maintaining an erection. They may simply give up before or during sexual activity because of shortness of breath or associated frustration. Women may just have less interest in general or may fail to 'turn on' to the notion of sex or to appropriate suggestions by her partner.

(1984: 117–18)

Thus Kass *et al.* (1972), for example, reported that 19 per cent of their male COAD patients were impotent, whilst more recent studies have suggested higher rates of sexual dysfunction amongst men. Fletcher and Martin (1982), for instance, reported that 30 per cent of their COAD patients were impotent and that an additional 5 per cent had ceased sexual intercourse due to dyspnoea. As they conclude:

Data from this study suggest that sexual dysfunction and erectile impotence can accompany COPD in the absence of other known causes of sexual problems. Furthermore, sexual dysfunction tended to be worse in those subjects with more severe pulmonary function impairment as assessed by pulmonary function tests, blood gases, and exercise tests.

(Quoted in McSweeny and Labuhn 1990: 401)

Only limited data exist regarding sexual dysfunction in female COAD sufferers. In Hanson's (1982) study (62 per cent male; 38 per cent female), for example, it was found that amongst the eleven areas assessed, sexual functioning was the one most consistently rated as having been negatively affected by COAD. Unfortunately, however, Hanson did not provide an analysis of these results by gender. Also, in another interesting study, Sexton and Monro (1985) found that wives of male COAD sufferers reported significantly lower levels of sexual intercourse compared to age-matched controls. Indeed, some 54 per cent of wives, compared to 15 per cent of controls, stated that they had no desire for sexual relations. These wives also gave significantly lower ratings on their perceived health status, which may account for this finding, although, as discussed earlier, lower health status may itself be related to the caring role (McSweeny and Labuhn 1990).

As McSweeny and Labuhn (1990) note, although the sexual functioning of female COAD sufferers remains a relatively neglected area, it is probably safe to assume that the same factors which affect sexual functioning in men similarly affect women. Hence they conclude:

> [COAD] has a documented negative effect on sexual functioning in men and probably in women as well. Although psychosocial factors play an important role in sexual functioning, the sexual dysfunctioning associated with [COAD] is closely linked with cardiopulmonary dysfunction and hypoxemia.
>
> (1990: 402)

These findings find further support in Williams' (1990) recent study. COAD sufferers were asked whether their illness either currently or in the past had caused any problems with their sex lives. Seventy-six per cent stated that it had. Thus Mr O'Riley, when asked about his sex life, responded as follows:

Mr O'Riley: Oh, that's a thing of the past that is.

Interviewer: Why is that?

Mr O'Riley: That's down to me health, it's completely nothing, with me anyway, that's finished … it's non-existent … you have the interest all right, but there's no way, especially when you can't breathe, it's the breathlessness that finishes me, that's number one …

Interviewer: What sort of effect has that had on you?

Mr O'Riley: Well I don't know really how you'd explain it. It makes me feel like, ah [pause, sighs], it makes me feel useless, put it that way. I think that I'm useless, that I'm only a burden, and, ah, I can't do nothing anyway, either way. I can't do no work and me sex life, that's finished, has been for about ah [pauses]. So what am I, I'm just a cabbage, you know, that's the way I feel, the way I look at it sometimes now.

Mrs Prout, meanwhile, when asked whether the illness had affected her sex life, stated:

It has in the last two or three years or so. We always had a very good sex life and I don't love him [husband] any the less, it's nothing like that, you know. But I feel that I don't want to have intercourse any more, I seem to have lost interest in sex and I felt I was being unfair to him. I wasn't the type to have a 'headache' or anything like that, you know, but he's very understanding. It's only happened in the last two or three years, it hasn't been as it should be, and I've talked to him about it, 'cause you know, it worries me. Because it's all part of being married and having a good relationship, and we've always had a very good relationship. And I thought, 'Well, maybe it will sort of come back', but it never really has done, not fully. So that worries me, but he's been very understanding about it.

In addition to sexual dysfunction, chronic illness and disability may also, of course, pose considerable problems and difficulties with respect to child-bearing, child-rearing and performance of the parental role (Locker 1983). In this respect, COAD sufferers may fare better than, say, the rheumatoid arthritis or multiple sclerosis sufferer, as the condition predominantly tends to occur in middle to later life when the parental role is nearing completion and the children have grown up. The majority of those in Williams' (1990) study, for instance, claimed that their illness and disability had not caused any real problems or difficulties with respect to their own children. Indeed, if anything, it was grown-up children who were now, in varying degrees, providing help and support for their parents. Instead, most of the accounts given centred upon the fact that sufferers were unable to perform the *grand*parental role to the extent they wished or desired, and of the feelings surrounding this and the upset it generated. Thus as Mr Thomas stated:

I sit here and I look at that photo of her [granddaughter] up there and I think to myself, 'If only I was all right what would I be doing with her now', probably playing with her or carting her off on holiday with us somewhere. You see, I can't even play with her, I can't pick her up, she's too heavy now, and I find that very upsetting and I do get a bit emotional about it at times, you know.

Similarly, concerning things which were missed, Mr and Mrs Ash stated:

Mrs Ash: Not being able to play with his granddaughter a bit more.

Mr Ash: Yeah, 'cause I used to enjoy playing with her and now I find
that I can't. If I play about with her too much it leaves me
breathless. Not being able to pick her up and play with her,
that upsets me.

Meanwhile Mrs McLeod, who had five grandchildren, spoke of how she
missed seeing and playing with them as much as she used to in the past:

I used to have them down to stay and I would play with them and all
that, you know, but I can't do it now. I mean, even when they do come
up now, they'll bring a game up and play, but after a while, I find I just
can't cope with it all, I start getting breathless. I mean I love 'em
dearly, but I just can't seem to cope with them for any length of time
now.

Again, however, this is not to suggest a wholly negative picture, for as
Hanson (1982) found in her study, some 28 per cent of COAD patients
indicated a positive gain in this area; presumably due to the abundance of
time available to see their grandchildren as a consequence of the illness.

In attempting to draw the diverse threads of this chapter together in
closing, it can readily be appreciated how the consequences of COAD
span a broad range of areas, aspects and dimensions of social, recreational
and family life. These include dwindling social and recreational lives;
social isolation; problems of social interaction, stigma, legitimacy and the
tolerance of others towards the condition; the threat or reality of
'dependency' and of being a 'burden' upon others; and, finally, problems
pertaining to sexuality and family life. Some of these issues are subtle and
intangible (i.e. what Bury [1988] terms 'meaning as *significance*'), others
are more concrete and overt (i.e. what Bury [1988] terms 'meaning as
consequence'), yet all are profoundly important influences not only upon
sufferers' and their families' quality of life, but also upon the images and
conceptions they hold of themselves and others. As Blaxter (1976)
suggests, it is problems and difficulties such as these which, for the
disabled, may prove to be the most distressing, intractable and difficult to
resolve and which, in large part, constitute the real *meaning of disability*.

Chapter 7

Conclusions and policy implications

As the previous chapters have attempted to convey, COAD sufferers and their families face a broad range of problems as a consequence of the disease. It should, however, be emphasised that many of the studies discussed within the course of this book, including the author's own study, are composed of either COAD out-patients or hospitalised in-patients. As such, these studies may not be representative of the COAD population as a whole, many of whom, due to the insidious nature of the disease process discussed in Chapters two and three, have yet to seek specialist medical help and treatment for their condition. Yet, given this caveat, the findings of these studies are probably fairly typical, in varying degrees, of the experience of COAD following the development and subsequent presentation of frank clinical illness.

We have seen, for example, the considerable distress which COAD and its associated symptomatology, particularly breathlessness, may bring in its wake (Chapter two); the nature and extent of disability which may accompany COAD, spanning a broad range of roles and activities of relevance to sufferers' quality of life, such as work, recreation and pastimes, household management, sleep and rest, ambulation and mobility (Chapter four); and, finally, the considerable vocational, financial, social and familial hardship or handicap (WHO 1980) which may accompany COAD (Chapters five and six). Moreover, it is also clear that psychosocial as well as physiological factors play an important role not only in relation to the experience and management of COAD as such, but also in terms of sufferers' disability and quality of life more generally. Hence, it is to the wider policy implications of these issues, not only for health care professionals working within this area, but also for health and welfare policy more generally, that this concluding chapter now turns. In this respect four main points emerge.

First, the slow and insidious nature of COAD's onset seems to suggest the need to target vulnerable groups (i.e. working-class, smokers, etc.) in terms of routine screening procedures such as simple spirometric measures of lung function, aimed at the early detection of the disease (i.e. a focus upon the early signs of underlying respiratory impairment) and the modification of established risk factors such as smoking. The efficacy of such an approach is further highlighted by evidence which suggests that it is only by bringing to the attention of these vulnerable groups the *actual* manifestations of disease, *vis-à-vis* the *potential* health risks associated with such behaviours, that changes in health-risking behaviours such as smoking actually occur (Calnan and Williams 1991). At present, the tragic fact still remains that, all too often, by the time the disease is clinically presented, irreversible damage has already been done. It is to be hoped that the recent emphasis upon health promotion and disease prevention within the new GP contract will serve to encourage the routine adoption of such a strategy by primary health care teams.

Second, it is also clear that 'quality of life is not simply a function of the patient's cardiopulmonary pathophysiology' (McSweeny and Labuhn 1990: 411). Indeed, as has been emphasised throughout the course of this book, the important role of psychosocial as well as physiological factors in the experience of COAD, the patient's ability to cope with the disease and to benefit from treatment and rehabilitation, needs not only emphasising but also more fully exploiting (McSweeny and Labuhn 1990). Current research suggests that the patient with the poorest quality of life is least likely to respond to traditional interventions due to disease-associated features such as 'advanced age, low social position, depressed cognitive set and neuropsychological deficit' (McSweeny and Labuhn 1990: 412). Yet, as McSweeny and Labuhn note: 'The fact that there is an interrelationship between psychosocial and physiological factors in [COAD] has been exploited infrequently in the clinical situation' (1990: 410). Hence, it seems clear that psychosocial variables should be:

> included as outcome variables in most patients and as a predictor or moderator variables in some patients, when medical and rehabilitative interventions for [COAD] are being evaluated. In addition ... psychological factors may also be useful in explaining aspects of respiration in [COAD] that cannot otherwise be explained.
>
> (McSweeny and Labuhn 1990: 411)

It is in this respect that, as McSweeny and Labuhn (1990) themselves suggest, Engel's (1980) concept of a *biopsychosocial* model seems particularly appropriate for the treatment and management of COAD. In particular, those working with COAD sufferers and their families should possess good interpersonal skills, demonstrate time, willingness and ability to listen, and be able to offer help and advice on how best to cope not only with the bio-physical, but also the psychosocial sequelae of the disease and their mutually reinforcing nature; issues which have provided the main focus of this book. This may require a formal evaluation of psychosocial functioning as part of a comprehensive assessment of COAD patients covering patients' and, wherever possible, carers' emotional functioning, social role functioning, activities of daily living, sexuality, recreation and pastimes (see McSweeny and Labuhn [1990] for a useful discussion of relevant methods and instruments). As McSweeny and Labuhn (1990) suggest, once the assessment has been completed, an intervention plan specifically tailored to patients' (and carers') own particular needs should be developed. Some may be functioning well and require only simple advice and reassurance, whilst others may require considerable practical help and psychosocial support.

As we have seen, psychosocial issues may also, of course, be handled effectively in formal pulmonary rehabilitation programmes. As Dudley *et al.* (1980) suggest, a fruitful approach may be to integrate psychosocial supports into a multi-modal pulmonary rehabilitation programme covering, for instance, things such as routine medical management, breathing re-training and therapy, graduated exercise, group therapy sessions and voluntary counselling on psychosocial and vocational issues (see Chapter three).

Third, as discussed in Chapter five, the eligibility criteria regarding disablement benefits such as mobility and attendance allowance – subsumed from April 1992 under the new Disability Living Allowance – tend to be geared towards the more 'obvious' musculo-skeletal types of disability and 'traditional' ADL items, rather than the more subtle respiratory-related disabilities (Williams 1989a, b). Eligibility criteria for mobility allowance, for example, are both strict and narrow. Consequently, despite the often considerable degree of difficulty and distress involved, the majority of COAD sufferers can indeed still walk across the room or to the front gate; a fact which, unfortunately all too often, invalidates their application. Moreover, as I have argued elsewhere (Williams 1989a, b), this 'bias' also relates to and reflects a similar bias in many of the traditional disability indices which have hitherto been used in disablement research, particularly ADL-type scales. Hence, there is a need for the development of ever more sensitive measures of breathlessness, respiratory disability and quality of life impairment. The development of such instruments is important not only for the measurement of treatment benefits and the development of optimal care (Guyatt *et al.* 1987), but also in highlighting 'need' and entitlement to welfare benefits, particularly in the light of the often considerable financial disadvantage which may accompany COAD.

The fourth and final point concerns the specific issue of social disadvantage or handicap (WHO 1980). It seems clear that reductions within the wide range of areas of handicap documented within this book could bring about major improvements in the quality of life of COAD patients and their families, though one is mindful, of course, of the distress which persistent symptoms create under any circumstances (see Chapter two). This is to imply not that health care teams working within this area are altogether unaware of such issues; rather, that, at a general level, a more systematic policy for tackling these problems and issues seems called for; one which may well extend far beyond the medical care and rehabilitation setting and involve a closer liaison with other service providers (Bury 1979).

As we have seen, COAD represents one of a range of chronic conditions which has little appeal to public sentiments. Self-help activities also appear fairly limited in this area, partly as a result of the restrictions of the disability involved, and partly as a result of issues pertaining to the stigma and legitimacy of the condition. COAD's association with deprived occupational and social circumstances further reinforces this view. Moreover, the frequent reliance upon immediate family for care and social support throws into sharp relief the 'unremitting burden of carers' (Anderson 1987) which occurs 'behind closed doors'. This serves to warns us against placing too much emphasis upon informal 'community care' (Bulmer 1987). COAD patients and their families are thus in need of considerable help and support from formal (health) service providers. As Blaxter (1983) points out, this should equally concern the consequences of poverty as well as the management of symptoms. The concept of handicap or social disadvantage (WHO 1980), in particular, directs our attention to these wider social consequences of chronic illness which need to be at the forefront of any further development of services for COAD patients and their families.

References

Agle, D.F., Baum, G.L. and Chester, E.H. (1973) 'Multidiscipline treatment of chronic pulmonary insufficiency: psychologic aspects of rehabilitation', *Psychosomatic Medicine* 35: 41–9

American Lung Association (1975) *Report of the Task Force on Comprehensive and Continuing Care for Patients with Chronic Obstructive Pulmonary Disease*, New York: American Lung Association.

Anderson, R. (1987) 'The unremitting burden of carers', *British Medical Journal* 294: 73–4.

Anderson, R. (1988) 'The quality of life of stroke patients and their carers', in R. Anderson and M. Bury (eds) *Living with Chronic Illness: The Experience of Patients and Their Families*, London: Unwin Hyman.

Anderson, R. and Bury, M. (eds) (1988) *Living with Chronic Illness: The Experience of Patients and Their Families*, London: Unwin Hyman.

Badham, C. (1808) *Observations on the Inflammatory Affections of the Mucous Membrane of the Bronchiae*, London: Callow.

Barstow, R.E. (1974) 'Coping with emphysema', *Nursing Clinics of North America* 9: 137–45.

Baum, G.L., Agle, D.F. and Chester, E.H. (1973) 'Multidiscipline treatment of chronic pulmonary insufficiency: functional status at one-year follow up', in R.F. Johnson (ed.) *Pulmonary Care*, New York: Grune & Stratton.

Blane, D. (1985) 'An assessment of the Black Report's explanation of health inequalities', *Sociology of Health and Illness* 7: 423–45.

Blaxter, M. (1976) *The Meaning of Disability*, London: Heinemann.

Blaxter, M. (1983) 'Health services as a defence against the consequences of poverty in industrialised societies', *Social Science and Medicine* 17: 1139–48.

Blaxter, M. (1987) 'Health and social class: evidence on inequality in health from a national survey', *Lancet* i: 30–3.

Blaxter, M. (1990) *Health and Lifestyles*, London: Routledge.

Britten, N., Davies, J.M.C. and Colley, J.T.R. (1987) 'Early respiratory experience and subsequent cough and peak expiratory flow rate in 36-year-old men and women', *British Medical Journal* 2: 1317–20.

Bruhn, J. (1977) 'Effects of chronic illness on the family', *Journal of Family Practice* 4: 1057–60.

Bulmer, M. (1987) *The Social Basis of Community Care*, London: Allen & Unwin.

Bums, B.H. and Howell, J.B.L. (1969) 'Disproportionately severe breathlessness in chronic bronchitis', *Quarterly Journal of Medicine* 38: 277–94.

Burr, M.L., St Leger, A.S. and Yarnell, J.W.G. (1981) 'Wheezing, dampness and coal fires', *Community Medicine* 3: 205–9.

Burrows, B. (1985) 'Course and prognosis in advanced disease', in T.L. Petty (ed.) *Chronic Obstructive Pulmonary Disease* (2nd edn), New York: Marcel Dekker.

Burton, L. (1975) *The Family Life of Sick Children*, London: Routledge & Kegan Paul.

Bury, M. (1978) 'A cloak of mystery: social aspects of ankylosing spondylitis', paper given at the National Ankylosing Spondylitis Society Symposium, The King's Fund Centre, London, November.

Bury, M. (1979) 'Disablement in society: towards an integrated perspective', *International Journal on Rehabilitation Research* 2 (1): 33–40.

Bury, M. (1982) 'Chronic illness as biographical disruption', *Sociology of Health and Illness* 4 (2): 167–82.

Bury, M. (1988) 'Meanings at risk: living with rheumatoid arthritis', in R. Anderson and M. Bury (eds) *Living with Chronic Illness: The Experiences of Patients and Their Families*, London: Unwin Hyman.

Calnan, M. and Williams, S.J. (1991) 'Style of life and the salience of health: a study of health-related practices in middle-class and working-class households', *Sociology of Health and Illness* 13 (4): 506–29.

Capel, L.H. and Caplin, M. (1964) *Chronic Bronchitis in Great Britain*, London: The Heart and Chest Association.

Cassileth, B.R., Lusk, E.J. and Strouse, T.B. (1984) 'Psychosocial status in chronic illness: a comparative analysis of six diagnostic groups', *New England Journal of Medicine* 311: 506–10.

Charmaz, K. (1983) 'The loss of self: a fundamental form of suffering in the chronically ill', *Sociology of Health and Illness* 5: 168–95.

Colley, J.R.T., Douglas, J.W.B. and Reid, D.D. (1970) 'Urban and social origins of childhood bronchitis in England and Wales', *British Medical Journal* 2: 213.

Colley, J.R.T., Douglas, J.W.B. and Reid, D.D. (1973) 'Respiratory disease in young adults: influence of lower respiratory illness, social class, air pollution and smoking', *British Medical Journal* 3: 195–8.

Cornwell, J. (1984) *Hard-Earned Lives: Accounts of Health and Illness from East London*, London: Tavistock.

Darwin C. (1895/1955) *The Expression of Emotion in Man and Animals*, New York: Philosophical Library.

Dudley, D.L., Glaser, E.M., Jorgenson, B.N. and Logan, D.L. (1980) 'Psychosocial concomitants to rehabilitation in chronic obstructive pulmonary disease. Part 1: psychosocial and psychological considerations', *Chest* 77 (3): 413–20.

Dudley, D.L., Verhey, J.W. and Masuda, M. (1969) 'Long-term adjustment, prognosis and death in irreversible diffuse obstructive pulmonary syndromes', *Psychosomatic Medicine* 31: 310–25.

Dudley, D.L., Wermuth, C. and Hague, W. (1973) 'Psychosocial aspects of care in chronic obstructive pulmonary disease', *Heart and Lung* 2: 289–303.

Elias, N. (1978) *The Civilizing Process. Volume 1: The History of Manners*, Oxford: Basil Blackwell.

Engel, G. (1980) 'The clinical application of the biopsychosocial model', *American Journal of Psychiatry* 13: 535–43.

Fagerhaugh, S. (1975) 'Getting around with emphysema', in A.L. Strauss (ed.) *Chronic Illness and the Quality of Life*, St Louis, MO: Mosby.

Finch, J. and Groves, D. (eds) (1983) *A Labour of Love: Women, Work and Caring*, London: Routledge & Kegan Paul.

Fitzpatrick, R.M. (1984) 'Satisfaction with health care', in R. Fitzpatrick, J. Hinton, S. Newman, G. Scambler and J. Thompson, *The Experience of Illness*, London: Tavistock.

Fletcher, C.M., Elmes, P.C., Fairbairn, A.S. and Wood, C.H. (1959) 'The significance of respiratory symptoms and the diagnosis of chronic bronchitis in a working population', *British Medical Journal* 2: 257–66.

Fletcher, C.M., Peto, R., Tinker, C. and Speizer, F.E. (1976) *The Natural History of Chronic Bronchitis and Emphysema*, Oxford: Oxford University Press.

Fletcher, E.C. and Martin, R.J. (1982) 'Sexual dysfunction and erectile impotence in chronic obstructive pulmonary disease', *Chest* 81: 413–21.

Freidson, E. (1970) *The Profession of Medicine*, New York: Dodd Mead.

Goffman, E. (1963) *Stigma: Notes on the Management of Spoiled Identity*, Englewood Cliffs, NJ: Prentice Hall.

Goffman, E. (1971) 'The insanity of place', in E. Goffman, *Relations in Public: Microstudies of the Public Order*, London: Allen Lane.

Goldberg, D.P. and Huxley, P. (1980) *Mental Illness in the Community*, London: Tavistock.

Grant, I. and Heaton, R. (1985) 'Neuropsychiatric abnormalities', in T.L. Petty (ed.) *Chronic Obstructive Pulmonary Disease* (2nd edn), New York: Marcel Dekker.

Guyatt, G.H., Townsend, M., Berman, L.B. and Pugsley, S.O. (1987) 'Quality of life in patients with chronic airflow limitation', *British Journal of Disease of the Chest* 81: 45–54.

Hanson, E.I. (1982) 'The effects of chronic lung disease on life in general and on sexuality: perceptions of adult patients', *Heart and Lung* 11 (5): 435–41.

Harris, A.I., Cox, E. and Smith, C.R.W. (1971) *Handicapped and Impaired in Great Britain*, London: HMSO.

Hinton, J. (1967) *Dying*, Harmondsworth: Pelican.

Holma, B. and Kjaer, G. (1980) 'Alcohol, housing and smoking in relation to respiratory symptoms', *Environmental Research* 21: 126–42.

Hunter, D. (1975) *The Diseases of Occupations* (5th edn), London: English Universities Press.

Hunter, J. (1986) 'What does "virtually unable to walk" mean?' *British Medical Journal* 292: 172–3.

Jensen, P.S. (1983) 'Risk protective factors and supportive interventions in chronic airways obstruction', *Archives of General Psychiatry* 40: 1203–7.

Jones, P.W. (1988) 'Measuring the quality of life of patients with respiratory disease', in S.R. Walker and R. Rosser (eds) *Quality of Life: Assessment and Application*, Lancaster: MTP Press Ltd.

Kaptein, A.A. (1982) 'Psychosocial correlates of length of hospitalization and rehospitalization in patients with acute, severe asthma', *Social Science and Medicine* 16: 725–9.

Kass, I., Updegraff, K. and Muffly, R.B. (1972) 'Sex in chronic obstructive pulmonary disease', *Medical Aspects of Human Sex* 6: 33–42.

Kelleher, D. (1988) *Diabetes*, London: Routledge.

Kiernan, K.E., Colley, J.R.T., Douglas, J.W.B. and Reid, D.D. (1976) 'Chronic cough in young adults in relation to smoking habits, childhood environment and chest illness', *Respiration* 33: 236–44.

Kinsman, R.A., Yaroush, R.A., Fernandez, E., Dirks, J.F., Schocket, M. and Fukahara, J. (1983) 'Symptoms and experiences in chronic bronchitis and emphysema', *Chest* 83: 755–61.

Labuhn, K.T. (1984) 'An analysis of self-reported depressed mood in chronic obstructive pulmonary disease' (Doctoral Dissertation, University of Michigan, 1984), *Dissertation Abstracts International* 45: 524B.

Lane, D. (1988) 'Disabling breathlessness', in A.O. Frank and G.P. Maguire (eds) *Disabling Diseases*, London: Heinemann.

Lester, D.M. (1973) 'The psychological impact of chronic obstructive pulmonary disease', in R.F. Johnson (ed.) *Pulmonary Care*, New York: Grune & Stratton.

Locker, D. (1983) *Disability and Disadvantage: The Consequences of Chronic Illness*, London: Tavistock.

Logan, D.L. and Johnson, R.L., Jr. (1974) *Pulmonary SCOR Excerpts From Annual Progress Reports, National Heart and Lung Institute*, National Institutes of Health, USA, 1 March.

Lustig, F.M., Haas, A. and Castillo, R. (1972) 'Clinical and rehabilitation regime in patients with COPD', *Archives of Physical Medicine and Rehabilitation* 53: 315–22.

MacIntyre, S. (1986) 'The patterning of health by social position in contemporary Britain: directions for sociological research', *Social Science and Medicine* 23: 393–415.

MacIntyre, S. (1988) 'A review of the social patterning and significance of measures of height, weight, blood pressure and respiratory function', *Social Science and Medicine* 27 (4): 327–38.

McGavin, C.R., Gupta, G.P. and McHardy, G.J.R. (1976) 'Twelve minute walking test for assessing disability in chronic bronchitis', *British Medical Journal* 1: 822–3.

McGavin, C.R., Artvinli, M., Naoe, H. and McHardy G.J.R. (1978) 'Dyspnoea, disability and distance walked: a comparison of estimates of exercise performance in respiratory disease', *British Medical Journal* 2: 241–3.

McSweeny, A.J., Grant, I., Heaton, R.K., Adams, K.M. and Timms, R.M. (1982) 'Life quality of patients with chronic obstructive pulmonary disease', *Archives of Internal Medicine* 142: 473–8.

McSweeny, A.J. and Labuhn, K.T. (1990) 'Chronic obstructive pulmonary disease', in B. Spilker (ed.) *Quality of Life Assessment in Clinical Trials*, New York: Raven Press Ltd.

Mausner, J.S. (1970) 'Cigarette smoking among patients with respiratory disease', *American Review of Respiratory Disease* 102: 704–13.

Meadows, S.H. (1961) 'Social class migration and chronic bronchitis', *British Journal of Social Medicine* 15: 171–6.

Medical Research Council Committee on the Aetiology of Chronic Bronchitis (MRC) (1965) 'Definitions and classification of chronic bronchitis for clinical and epidemiological purposes', *Lancet* i: 775.

Morgan, A.D., Peck, D.F., Buchanan, D.R. and McHardy, G.J.R. (1983a) 'Effect of attitudes and beliefs on exercise tolerance in chronic bronchitis', *British Medical Journal* 286: 171–3.

Morgan, A.D., Peck, D.F., Buchanan D.R. and McHardy, G.J.R. (1983b) 'Psychological factors contributing to disproportionate disability in chronic bronchitis', *Journal of Psychosomatic Research* 27: 259–61.

Morgan, M., Calnan, M. and Manning, N. (1985) *Sociological Approaches to Health and Medicine*, London: Croom Helm.

Moroney, R. (1976) *The Family and the State*, New York: Longman.

Nocon, A. and Booth, T. (1991) 'The social impact of asthma', *Family Practice* 8 (1): 37–41.

Office of Health Economics (OHE) (1977) *Preventing Bronchitis*, London: OHE.

Office of Population Censuses and Surveys (OPCS) (1988a) *The Prevalence of Disability Among Adults*, London: HMSO.

Office of Population Censuses and Surveys (OPCS) (1988b) *The Financial Circumstances of Disabled Adults Living in Private Households*, London: HMSO.

Patrick, D.L. and Peach, H. (eds) (1989) *Disablement in the Community*, Oxford: Oxford University Press.

Pederson L.L. (1982) 'Compliance with physician advice to quit smoking: a review of the literature', *Preventive Medicine* 11: 71–84.

Petty, T.L. (ed.) (1985) *Chronic Obstructive Pulmonary Disease* (2nd edn), New York: Marcel Dekker.

Petty, T.L. (1988) 'Medical management of COPD', in A.J. McSweeny and I. Grant (eds) *Chronic Obstructive Pulmonary Disease: A Behavioral Perspective*, New York: Marcel Dekker.

Petty, T.L. and Nett, L.M. (1984) *Enjoying Life with Emphysema*, Philadelphia, PA: Lea & Febiger.

Prigatano, G.P. and Grant, I. (1988) 'Neuropsychological correlates of COPD', in A.J. McSweeny and I. Grant (eds) *Chronic Obstructive Pulmonary Disease: A Behavioral Perspective*, New York: Marcel Dekker.

Prigatano, G.P., Wright, E.C. and Levine D. (1984) 'Quality of life and its predictors in patients with mild hypoxemia and chronic obstructive pulmonary disease', *Archives of Internal Medicine* 144: 1613–19.

Robinson, I. (1988) *Multiple Sclerosis*, London: Routledge.

Rosser, R. and Guz, A. (1981) 'Psychological treatments for breathlessness', *Journal of Psychosomatic Research* 25: 439–47.

Rosser, R., Denford, J., Heslop, A., Kinston, W., Macklin, D., Minty, K., Moynihan, C., Muir, B., Rein, L. and Guz, A. (1983) 'Breathlessness and psychiatric morbidity in chronic bronchitis and emphysema: a study of psychotherapeutic management', *Psychological Medicine* 13: 93–110.

Royal College of Physicians of London (RCP) (1981) 'Disabling chest disease: prevention and care', *Journal of the Royal College of Physicians of London* 15 (2): 69–87.

Rubeck, M.F. (1971) *Social and Emotional Effects of Chronic Bronchitis*, London: The Chest and Heart Association.

Rutter, B.M. (1977) 'Some psychological concomitants of chronic bronchitis', *Psychological Medicine* 7: 459–64.

Rutter, B.M. (1979) 'The prognostic significance of psychological factors in the management of chronic bronchitis', *Psychological Medicine* 9: 63–70.

Scadding, J.G. (1981) 'Talking clearly about broncho-pulmonary diseases', in J.G. Scadding and G. Cumming (eds) *Scientific Foundations of Respiratory Medicine*, London: Heinemann Medical Books Ltd.

Scambler, G. (1989) *Epilepsy*, London: Routledge.

Schudson M. (1984) 'Embarrassment and Erving Goffman's idea of human nature', *Theory and Society* 13: 633–48.

Sexton, D.L. and Monro, B.H. (1985) 'Impact of a husband's chronic illness (COPD) on the spouse's life', *Research in Nursing and Health* 8: 83–90.

Sexton, D.L. and Monro, B.H. (1988) 'The experience of women with chronic obstructive pulmonary disease (COPD)', *Western Journal of Nursing Research* 10: 26–44.

Shearer, A. (1981) *Disability: Whose Handicap?*, Oxford: Basil Blackwell.

Solzhenitsyn, A. (1968) *A Day in the Life of Ivan Denisovich*, Harmondsworth: Penguin.

Sontag, S. (1978) *Illness as Metaphor*, Harmondsworth: Penguin.

Stollenwerk, R. (1985) 'An emphysema client: self-care', *Home Healthcare Nurse* 3: 36–40.

Strauss, A.L. (1975) *Chronic Illness and the Quality of Life*, St Louis, MO: Mosby.

Tockman, M.S., Khoury M.J. and Cohen B.H. (1985) 'The epidemiology of COPD', in T.L. Petty (ed.) *Chronic Obstructive Pulmonary Disease* (2nd edn), New York: Marcel Dekker

Townsend, P. (1979) *Poverty in the United Kingdom*, Harmondsworth: Penguin.

Townsend, P., Davidson, N. and Whitehead, M. (1988) *Inequalities in Health: The Black Report and the Health Divide*, Harmondsworth: Penguin.

Walker, A. (1981) 'Disability and income', in A. Walker and P. Townsend (eds) *Disability in Britain: A Manifesto of Rights*, Oxford: Martin Robertson.

Weiner C. (1975) 'The burden of rheumatoid arthritis: tolerating the uncertainty', *Social Science and Medicine* 9: 97–104.

West, P. (1989) 'Income, work, and disability', in D.L. Patrick and H. Peach (eds) *Disablement in the Community*, Oxford: Oxford University Press.

Williams, S.J. (1989a) 'Chronic respiratory illness and disability: a critical review of the psychosocial literature', *Social Science and Medicine* 28: 791–803.

Williams, S.J. (1989b) 'Assessing the consequences of chronic respiratory disease: a critical review', *International Disability Studies* 11: 161–6.

Williams, S.J. (1990) 'The consequences of chronic respiratory illness: a sociological study', Unpublished Ph.D. thesis, University of London.

Williams, S.J. and Bury, M.R. (1989a) 'Impairment, disability and handicap in chronic respiratory illness', *Social Science and Medicine* 29 (5): 609–16.

Williams, S.J. and Bury, M.R. (1989b) '"Breathtaking": the consequences of chronic respiratory disorder', *International Disability Studies* 11: 114–20.

World Health Organisation (WHO) (1980) *International Classification of Impairments, Disabilities and Handicaps*, Geneva: WHO.

Young, R.F. (1982) 'Marital adaptation and response in chronic illness: the case of COPD' (Doctoral Dissertation, Wayne State University, 1981), *Dissertation Abstracts International* 42: 4947A.

Zola, I.K. (1973) 'Pathways to the doctor: from person to patient', *Social Science and Medicine* 7: 677–87.

Name index

Subject index